# Materia Medica
### granule
### potency
### apis
# Homeopathy
### testing
## constitution
### susceptibility

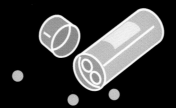

**Jean-Jacques Salva**
**Florence Portell**

CASSELL&CO

# 'Almost all men die from their cures and not from their illnesses!'

exclaimed Béralde in Molière's *The Hypochondriac*. When Christian Samuel Hahnemann discovered homeopathy at the end of the 18th century, conventional western medicine was primitive and needed development.

 20

**Since its discovery, over two centuries ago, homeopathy has provoked much controversy, criticism and impassioned support.**

 15

*Homeopathy is a system of complementary medicine which aims to treat each particular individual.*

*It represents real medical ecology. It is non-toxic and, when properly administered, does no harm to the body; it is also non-invasive and works to help the body's own healing powers.*

 16

# 'Like treats like'

Homeopathy uses medicines prepared from natural substances that are 'similar to the illness', unlike conventional medicine (known as **allopathy**) which treats and often suppresses the patient's symptoms.

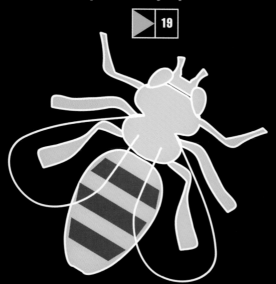

▶ | 19

*A woman came to my surgery having been stung by a swarm of bees, she was very red and swollen. Like any doctor, I immediately prepared a cortisone injection. However I noticed that the patient had no respiratory problems, which would have been the only reason for urgent intervention. Then I thought of Apis, the homeopathic medicine based on bee dilution.*

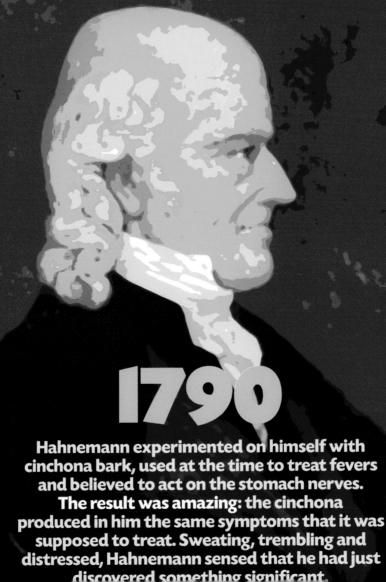

# 1790

Hahnemann experimented on himself with cinchona bark, used at the time to treat fevers and believed to act on the stomach nerves. The result was amazing: the cinchona produced in him the same symptoms that it was supposed to treat. Sweating, trembling and distressed, Hahnemann sensed that he had just discovered something significant.

# 1813

*Returning from the Russian campaign, Napoleon's armies have withdrawn to Leipzig.* They have brought with them **typhus** and **cholera** *which traditional doctors are powerless to control. However, using homeopathy, Hahnemann obtains results.*

## By the early 19th century

a Leipzig veterinary surgeon was already making homeopathic medicines which he administered to horses and cattle. Fifty years later, Dr Dehecq developed a homeopathic medicine to help animals give birth without difficulty.

**In his day**, *Hahnemann developed his own dilutions and medicines. His immediate successors did the same.* **Nowadays**, *most homeopathic medicines are manufactured in pharmaceutical laboratories according to strictly controlled procedures.*

A homeopathic prescription costs the NHS on average less than £2.

▷ 116

Approximately **3,500** vegetable, animal, mineral or chemical substances are used in the manufacture of homeopathic medicines.

▷ 72

An individual's constitution is the sum of all the elements which characterise him at any given moment in his life: family background, medical history, living conditions, physical and psychological environment.

▷ 71

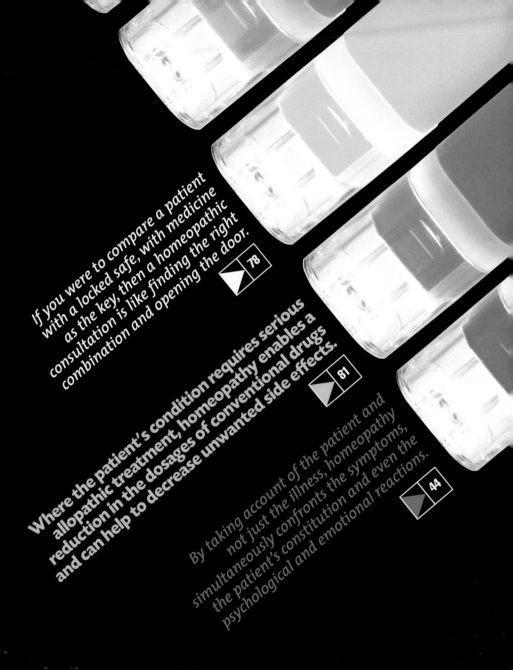

If you were to compare a patient with a locked safe, with medicine as the key, then a homeopathic consultation is like finding the right combination and opening the door. **78**

Where the patient's condition requires serious allopathic treatment, homeopathy enables a reduction in the dosages of conventional drugs and can help to decrease unwanted side effects. **81**

By taking account of the patient and not just the illness, homeopathy simultaneously confronts the symptoms, the patient's constitution and even the psychological and emotional reactions. **44**

**21** days to produce a mother tincture, **12** days to manufacture a globule and **16** days to manufacture a granule.

 116

**C** In centesimal dilutions, one drop of substance is mixed with 99 drops of solvent to obtain a dilution of 1c.

▶ 73

The lower the dilution, the greater its local effect on an acute condition and on a **physical** level.
The higher the dilution, the better its general effect on a chronic condition and on a **psychological** level.

▶ 74

*As a general rule, the more acute and recent the illness, the quicker it is cured by homeopathy.*

 77

Homeopathic medicines contain such low dilutions of
the mother tincture that,
according to conventional
chemistry, there is hardly a
molecule of the original active
constituent remaining in the
medicine.

▷ 24

**'Is homeopathy a placebo?'**
**If so, how can we explain that the therapy works not only on humans, who can be influenced psychologically, but also on plants and animals?**

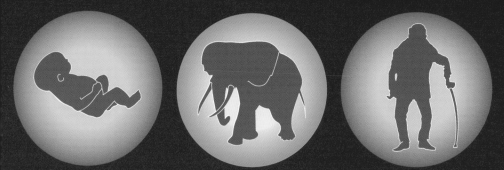

Using the same number of tablets, we can treat *an elephant or a mouse, an infant or an elderly person, since there is no real link between the amount of medicine taken and its effectiveness.*

Over the counter sales of homeopathic medicine *are growing by 20 per cent each year in Britain. 25 per cent of Scottish GPs have some homeopathic training.*

**Homeopathy is a fundamentally ecological practice:** the environment, which is polluted by antibiotics contained in human or animal waste, is unharmed in the case of homeopathic treatments which do not generate such waste.

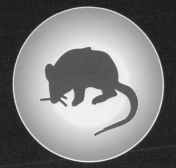

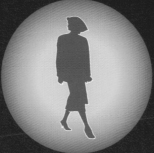

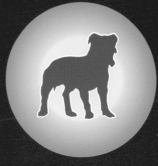

*Coffea,* the homeopathic medicine based on coffee dilution *treats shaking, agitation and insomnia, symptoms similar to those experienced by the coffee drinker.*

For stiff joints in the morning, made worse by cold, damp weather *but which improve during the day, 1 tablet of Rhus tox. 12c on getting up and during the day when pain occurs will help ease the joints and lift morale.*

***The consultation:*** *a homeopath asks questions that may seem remote from your problem but that enable him to work out your constitution, your susceptibility and your responses.*

 112

## Most people have their strengths and weaknesses. In homeopathy the goal is to consider the whole situation of which the ailment or weakness is a part. To do this, homeopaths try to identify the constitutional type of the patient.

68

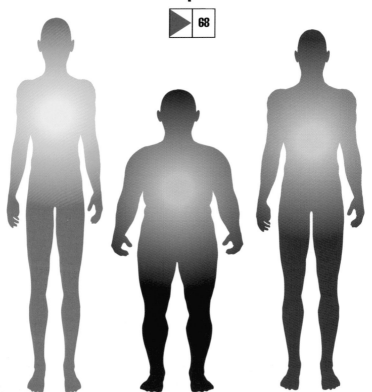

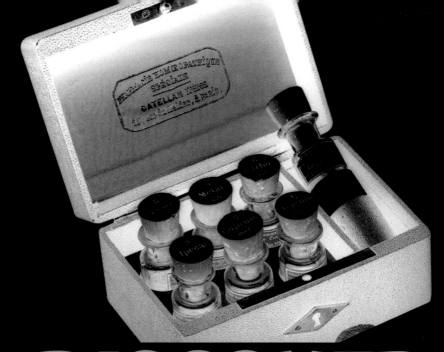

# DISCOVER

AT THE END OF THE 18TH CENTURY, A YOUNG GERMAN DOCTOR CALLED SAMUEL HAHNEMANN TOOK ADVANTAGE OF THE LATEST SCIENTIFIC DISCOVERIES OF HIS DAY TO RE-EXAMINE THE OLD SAYING, 'LIKE TREATS LIKE'. AS A RESULT OF HIS RESEARCH, HOMEOPATHY WAS BORN. IT HAS PROVOKED CRITICISM AND ARGUMENT BUT HAS NEVERTHELESS PROVED ITS EFFECTIVENESS. TODAY IT CONTINUES TO DIVIDE OPINION BETWEEN THOSE WHO ARE ENTHUSIASTIC AND THOSE WHO ARE SCEPTICAL OF ITS CLAIMS.

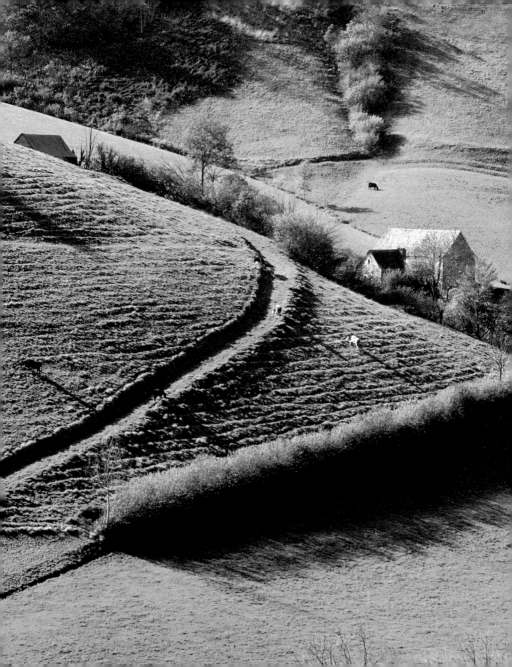

**S**ince its discovery over two centuries ago, no medical process has ever given rise to so much controversy, criticism or impassioned support. It is almost as if the theoretical debate has overshadowed the discussion of its therapeutic value. Homeopathy is the result of an experiment carried out by a German doctor, Samuel Hahnemann, who became disillusioned by the lack of discipline and scientific foundation for medicine as it was practised at the time. Homeopathy has come a long way since then and, like all genuine science, is still evolving. The following pages set out the main stages of its development, which have turned yesterday's medical discovery into a therapy perfectly adapted to tomorrow's world.

## MEDICAL COLLEGES AND TRAINING: FROM THEORY ...

Homeopathy is practised by medical doctors, other health care professionals and by homeo-paths – trained professionals who have studied at a variety of schools and have earned the right to add letters to their name indicating the qualifications they hold. In Britain these are likely to be LCHom, RSHom, UKHMA, MFHom, FFHom, LFHom (the last three being awarded to medical doctors). It is also worth noting that, in Britain, anyone can call them-selves a homeopath and set up in practice – always check qualifi-cations and preferably go by way of a recommendation or GP referral.

**MEDICINE IN THE COMMUNITY**

*When a doctor begins work in an everyday environment, the situation may be far removed from the sterile world of the hospital. With minimal equipment, he often practises in difficult circumstances.*

In the course of medical training, a doctor undertakes the study of a wide range of subjects: cardiology, rheumatology, surgery, psychiatry, gastroenterology and so on, before carrying out medical practice in a hospital or opting to work in the community as a general practitioner. However, before too long, it is likely that he or she will be confronted with a situation where it will be impossible to put into practice the methods that were taught in a clinical setting. It is difficult to take an X-ray by the roadside, for example, or set up a drip next to a patient confined to their bed at home. Or maybe a patient returns again and again with a chronic range of symptoms that do not respond to conventional drug treatment. The trainee doctor may begin to wonder about alternatives; listen to anecdotes from friends; read a few magazine articles; and finally go on to study a certified course in homeopathy.

## ... TO PRACTICE

'This is how homeopathic medicine came into my life as a doctor. I began by prescribing, as I thought appropriate, a remedy that I knew well. Just one! Little by little, I expanded my therapeutic tool kit. I always respected my patients' choices. I explained to my patients that I was training in homeopathy and suggested they try it with me. They always accepted and the results were often timely. Initially, I used homeopathy only for acute ailments such as fever, pain or rashes. Then, gradually, I included more general psychological problems. Finally, I used this method to approach constitutional problems like seasonal allergies or seasonal affective disorder and so on' (The experience of Dr Salva).

In fact, the homeopathic doctor has a very special way of getting to know the patient. He does not simply consider their symptoms, he also tries to work out how the patient 'lives' the illness. Homeopathy therefore becomes a way of helping people to recover their own particular equilibrium. It is a therapy which treats the individual, unlike orthodox medicine, where patients are grouped according to their symptoms. It does not harm the body, neither does it take over bodily function; rather it respects the integrity of the body and its own natural healing tendencies.

Doctors interested in homeopathy undertake postgraduate training following medical school. However, in Britain, homeopaths do not have to be medically qualified, although they do receive detailed medical knowledge as part of their specialised training. It is quite likely that practitioners will have decided to train as a homeopath as a result of experiencing a homeopathic cure or perhaps because they have seen a family member or friend apparently cured of a chronic complaint that did not respond to conventional treatment.

**A SICK CHILD**

*A raised temperature, weakness, hot flushes, sweating and thirst are indications for the prescription of* Belladonna *by a homeopath, the remedy is equally suitable for an adult or child.*

---

### SHOULD THE SYMPTOMS ALWAYS BE CONFRONTED?

---

Orthodox medicine is particularly concerned with symptoms and their suppression. Let's take the example of a mother who comes to the surgery because her child has a temperature of 40°C (104°F). The 'conventional' doctor usually prescribes an antipyretic drug based on aspirin or paracetamol to lower the temperature. However, this treatment fails to take account of an essential fact: the temperature is the body's best defence against infection, since it inhibits the spread of a virus. But does this matter, if the child's temperature falls as a result of this treatment and the mother is relieved? Unfortunately, it does matter because the virus seizes this opportunity and continues to spread. This weakens the body, making it vulnerable to further infection. The doctor then has to prescribe antibiotics, which will improve the situation until the end of the treatment. However, by doing the job that the body's immune system should have done, the drugs have prevented the body from manufacturing its own immunological defences. Such treatments actually leave the body weakened and increasingly vulnerable to bacterial attacks. After several such episodes, the mother is desperate because her child is pale and tired, with no appetite, and the child's school results are suffering. It is often in such circumstances that people go on to consult a homeopath.

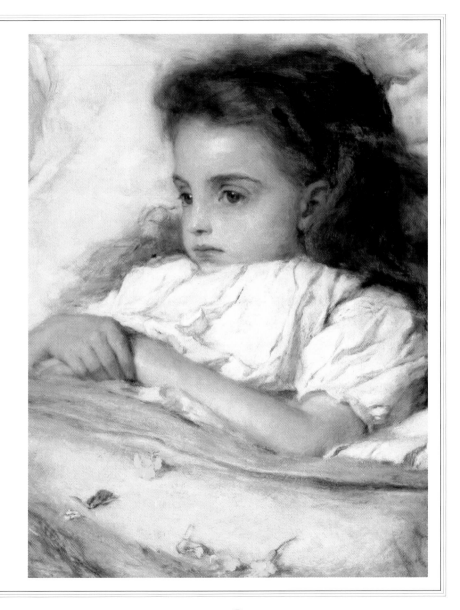

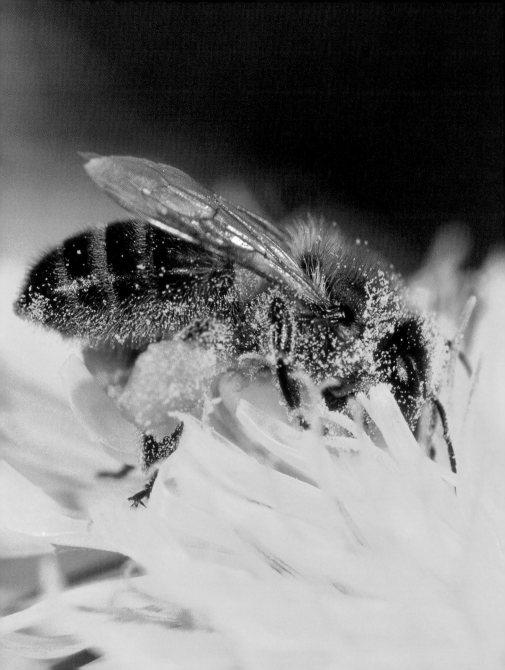

## APIS OR CORTISONE?

By seeking to help the patient's body defend itself, the homeopathic doctor tries to approach the problem differently. In the preceding example, the homeopath must find the medicine that corresponds not to fever in general, but to *this* precise fever as experienced by *this* particular child. When the body temperature drops, the child will be cured. The doctor, therefore, follows the advice of an old Chinese proverb: 'If you want to help a hungry man, don't give him a fish, give him a fishing rod and teach him to fish.'

**APIS MELLIFICA**

*To manufacture this remedy, the entire bee is soaked in an alcoholic solution.*

'I remember one of the first occasions when I was faced with a therapeutic dilemma, a woman came to my surgery with very red and swollen skin. She had just been stung by a swarm of bees. Like any doctor, I immediately prepared a cortisone injection. However, I noticed that the patient was experiencing no respiratory problems – these would normally indicate an allergic reaction and so the need for urgent intervention. Then I thought of *Apis*, the homeopathic medicine based on bee dilution. A very powerful anti-inflammatory, it seemed to me perfectly suited to this case. I suggested she try it. She agreed fairly readily since she was already familiar with homeopathy. Being a novice, keeping the cortisone injection ready in case of emergency, I administered *Apis* and then observed her closely for a moment. To my great surprise, the swelling began to go down visibly and within a few minutes the woman looked almost normal again. I must confess that as a precaution, I nevertheless gave her the cortisone injection before letting her leave. Nowadays, I would have confidence in the immediate effect of the medicine and I would no longer act in this way' (The experience of Dr Salva).

## LIKE TREATS LIKE

Homeopathy was developed in the late 18th and early 19th centuries by a German doctor, Christian Samuel Friedrich Hahnemann. The term, homeopathy, is made up of the Greek words *homoios*, meaning 'like', and *pathos*, meaning 'illness'. It is thus a method of medical treatment that uses substances which are 'like the illness', unlike conventional medicine which is known as allopathy from the Greek *allos*, meaning 'other', which treats an illness by using drugs which work against the disease and its symptoms. Hahnemann was not the first person to have noted the existence of what he called 'the law of similars'. More than two thousand years before him, the Greek doctor Hippocrates had already observed that *Cantharis*, while capable of curing common cystitis, could cause urinary irritation in a healthy subject. *Similia similibus curantur* ('like treats like') therefore sums up the law of similars that has been known for centuries. Hahnemann was born in Saxony in 1755 into a modest family where the twin principles of strictness and tolerance prevailed. His outstanding intelligence and appetite for work, encouraged several eminent people to provide him with financial support, which enabled him to undertake his medical studies in several universities. Equipped with a solid Graeco-Latin cultural background and fluent in German, French, English and Italian, the young Samuel earned his living translating works of chemistry and medicine.

Hahnemann was disheartened by medicine as it was practised at the time. 'Doctors are strange,' he wrote, 'they use remedies they know nothing about and administer them to bodies they know even less about.' Medical treatments of the time were based on imprecise clinical observations and included bloodletting and the use of leeches, as well as drugs such as mercury, which were toxic to the patient. Medicine had hardly advanced since a century earlier, when Molière had given Béralde the following line in his play *The Hypochondriac*: 'Almost all men die from their cures and not from their illnesses.'

**A GERMAN APOTHECARY IN THE 17TH CENTURY**

*At that time medicines were prepared using standard recipes, but there were no methods of testing remedies on patients.*

In 1777, driven by a keen desire for learning, Hahnemann left behind everything he knew to go to Vienna, then Europe's capital of arts and music. However, the city's joyful atmosphere hardly suited him. 'No!', he wrote, 'this is not what I came to find. I want to struggle with suffering and overcome pain.' At the age of 24, while working as a nurse in a psychiatric hospital, a job which included washing the sick and dressing their wounds, he successfully presented his doctoral thesis entitled 'Aetiology and treatment of spasmodic ailments', thus becoming a fully qualified doctor. He took an appointment as personal doctor to the governor of Transylvania, a post in which he spent nearly two years, enjoying a life of material comfort, short working hours and endless parties.

Paradoxically, what for others would have been a godsend, was considered by him to be a kind of punishment. 'I am sated with honours and wealth, whilst just a few kilometres away people are in agony. I am not a doctor. A doctor is something else. He is the man who relentlessly pursues sickness, struggling desperately against it, present at every bedside.'

### HAHNEMANN'S FRUSTRATION

Following a second visit to Vienna, Hahnemann settled in Dessau and made friends with a chemist, who, from time to time, allowed him to use his laboratory for his experiments. He married the chemist's adopted daughter, Henriette Kuchler, who bore him eleven children. However, Hahnemann was a perpetually dissatisfied man, who, despite often changing his place of residence, still found the local medical practices to be ineffective and unpleasant. 'They are poisoning people,' he wrote, 'they sell them sublimate and corrosives, give them arsenic, kill

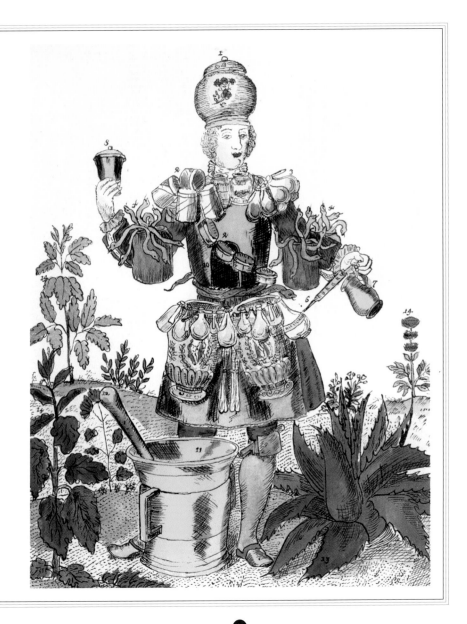

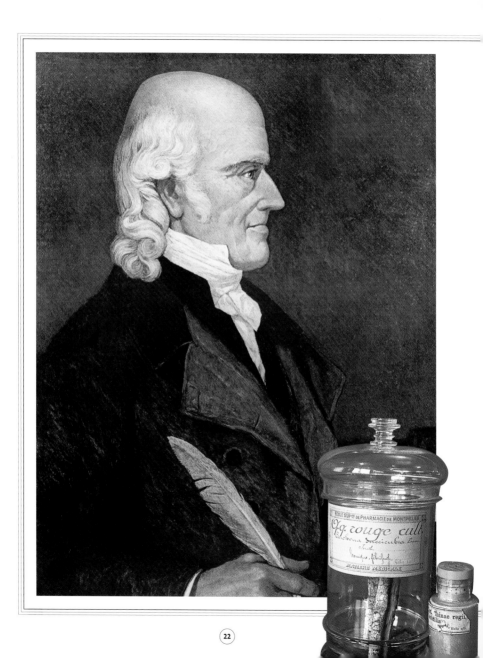

them through excessive bloodletting. Why?' His eventual rebellion against the medicine of his day coincided with the wind of revolution blowing through Europe which culminated in the French Revolution of 1789. In 1784, when Hahnemann was 29 years old, he could no longer tolerate his powerlessness when faced with the suffering of the sick. One day, after a child died in his arms, he decided to close his medical practice. To the great displeasure of his wife and family, he decided to devote himself to the research of more satisfactory therapeutic solutions. 'There is something to be found and it's staring us in the face,' he wrote, 'God did not forget to give us what we need to fight disease, it's not possible.'

**HAHNEMANN AND CINCHONA**

*With the discovery of the effects of cinchona (the homeopathic remedy known as China) on himself, Hahnemann pioneered the principle of experimentation that was to guide his future research.*

From then on, Hahnemann divided his time between the reading that sustained his research and the work he did as a translator that provided for his family. He was interested in the work of Hippocrates. 'We were never nearer to discovering the healing art than during the time of Hippocrates,' he wrote. 'This scrupulous observer sought to find the truth about health and disease. He described illnesses exactly, adding nothing, avoiding artistic licence and discussion. No doctor has since surpassed his talent for pure observation.' Hahnemann also studied Paracelsus and his 'signature theory' which was very fashionable at the time. This 16th-century alchemist-doctor had pushed the principle of similarity, described by Hippocrates, to its limits. In his opinion, the appearance of each plant indicated the illnesses it could cure: thus turmeric, a yellow spice, could cure jaundice; the flowers of St John's Wort, which produce a red sap, were able to heal bleeding wounds and so on. 'I am putting all these trivialities to one side,' wrote Hahnemann, although traces of them can sometimes still be found in the most recent reference works.

## THE INITIAL DISCOVERY

Interested in how some of these remedies worked, Hahnemann sought to understand matters in depth. In 1790 he translated an article written by an English doctor, William Cullen, on the subject of cinchona bark, widely used at the time to treat intermittent fevers accompanied by shaking, such as malaria. It was believed that the effect of cinchona was due to its action on the stomach nerves. 'There is one easy way to find out if it's true,' Hahnemann said to himself. 'Take the cure without being ill and study its effects.' The result astonished him, cinchona produced in him the same effects that it was supposed to treat. Sweating, shaking, distressed, Hahnemann sensed that he had just discovered something significant. What he didn't know was that fate had given him a helping hand, since not everyone is sensitive to cinchona in this way. He repeated his experiment using other substances and called upon the assistance of his close relations. His conviction grew that to treat 'like with like' was the pathway to discovering how to make a product which, in a healthy person, produces the same symptoms as those shown by the patient. It was this first experimentation that gave rise to the founding principle of homeopathy, a therapy based on the law of similars.

To improve the process of observing and classifying remedies, Hahnemann studied the work of other doctors of his time, including that of the French botanist François Boissier de Sauvages and the Briton, Edward Jenner, who was investigating cowpox inoculation. Jenner had established that inoculations containing the secretions from lesions caused by cowpox, a minor skin disease affecting cattle, could provide protection against smallpox in humans. This was the first example of vaccination in medical history. Hahnemann would later write, in the fourth edition of his classic text, the *Organon of the Healing Art*: 'Is it possible that cowpox provides protection from smallpox in any way other than homeopathically? It causes an illness very similar to cowpox, is therefore homeopathic, and having run its course, the human body which, as a rule, can only be affected once by an illness of this type, is then safe from any similar infection.' In 1796 he finally published his first essay in the *Journal of practical medicine and surgery*, a respected medical journal published in Germany by Doctor Hufeland, professor in pharmacology, member of the Academy of Science and doctor to the king of Prussia. This text, entitled 'Essay on a new principle for discovering the healing properties of medicinal substances', can be described as the birth certificate of homeopathy. 'All that remains,' wrote Hahnemann, 'is to test on the human body the medicines whose curative powers we wish to understand.'

## THE THEORY OF DILUTION

For around fifty years Hahnemann tested more than a hundred remedies of all kinds on himself and his friends and relations. However, one problem remained: the toxicity of certain substances used as remedies. For centuries poisons had been used as treatments to purge the body, occasionally giving rise to fatal accidents, as can well be imagined. Hahnemann had an idea that would become the second basic principle of homeopathy: reduce the doses of the remedies until all toxic risk was eliminated. And so he repeatedly reduced the remedy until it was dilute in the extreme. This was how the principle of infinitesimal doses was born. Homeopathic treatments use such low dilutions that, according to conventional chemical thinking, there is barely a molecule of the original active element remaining in the medicine. It has been suggested, however, that homeopathy functions as if a 'piece of

**JENNER AND COWPOX**

*Around 1790 the Briton Jenner discovered that inoculation of the cowpox vaccine allowed a healthy person to be protected against catching smallpox.*

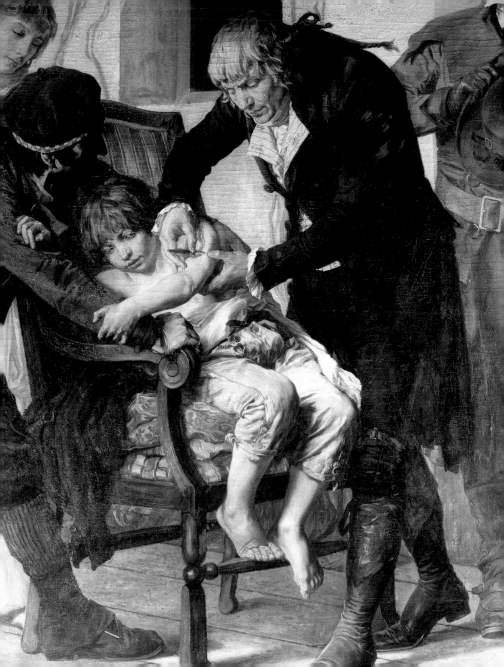

information' of an electromagnetic nature remains within the solvent and is thus transmitted to the patient taking it. In the late 20th century scientific work seemed to show at last that there might be some factual basis to this hypothesis.

Hahnemann was interested in the individual's predisposition to developing a particular illness as a result of constitutional weaknesses or any specific sensitivities and it was thus that the notion of susceptibility was born. This clarifies the notion of chronic miasmic illness, or diathesis: that is, the way in which successive illnesses occur in the same person. Two cornerstones of homeopathic theory were thus established and a completely new concept of the individual as a holistic being was realised through the study of the individual reactions of the patient during an episode of sickness.

In 1810, in Dresden, Germany, the first edition of the *Organon of the Healing Art* appeared, drawing together Hahnemann's ideas on medicine and setting out his methodology. This homeopathic reference work would later appear in six different editions in Germany (an exceptional achievement at the time), some of which would be translated into other languages. In 1811 the

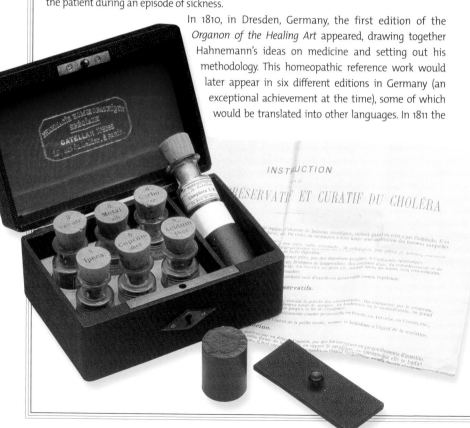

first volume of *Materia Medica Pura* was released, of which the sixth and last volume would be published in 1821. The second edition appeared in 1822.

By then, homeopathy was causing great excitement as people heard about the efficacy of the treatment and the sick arrived in large numbers at Hahnemann's surgery. In 1813 Napoleon's armies, returning from the Russian campaign, arrived in Leipzig, bringing with them typhus and cholera. The orthodox doctors were powerless to halt the scourge, but homeopathy obtained results. As a consequence, Hahnemann's reputation grew despite the fact that the medical community frowned at this alternative practitioner who propagated his controversial theories and even – a cardinal sin – made his own medicines!

### MATERIA MEDICA

In 1834, following the death of his wife, Hahnemann settled in the small town of Koethen. He lived with his daughter and continued to put the finishing touches to his work on homeopathy. At 79 years of age, he may have thought that fate would let him rest a little, but one day a young French woman arrived on his doorstep. Her name was Mélanie d'Hervilly and she was barely thirty. She was suffering from bronchitis and Hahnemann treated her, cured her and then married her. The couple settled in Paris in June 1835, at 26 rue des Saints-Pères. Almost immediately people started to flock to his clinic, especially after the publication of a report on his work in the *Krankenjournal (Journal of the Sick)* and the translation into French of his main works. Some well-meaning, but doubtful doctors protested and there were attempts to ban homeopathy. 'I'm not surprised,' observed Hahnemann, good-humouredly. 'If everything had suddenly become straightforward, I would have thought that God had abandoned me.'

**HOMEOPATHY AND CHOLERA**

*In 1813 Hahnemann cured Napoleon's soldiers from cholera. Almost two hundred years later homeopathy would be used again to treat this disease during an epidemic in South America.*

François Guizot, the French minister for public education, retorted to the protestors who were bombarding him: 'If homeopathy is a passing fad, it will die out of its own volition. If, on the other hand, it is a step forward for mankind, it will withstand all opposition and that is what the Academy (of Science) must hope for, in its mission to encourage discoveries.'

Hahnemann died in 1843 at the age of 88. On his death bed he bequeathed to his wife, Mélanie, the task of furthering his work. 'No one must follow my coffin,' he murmured, 'pride, that is the enemy.' In accordance with his wish, Mélanie took up the practice of homeopathy and continued to defend it against its opponents. She now lies by her husband's side in the Père-Lachaise cemetery in Paris and their tombs are maintained by the French Homeopathic Society.

During his long research career, Hahnemann tested the majority of products then used as medical treatments: animal matter (such as insects and venom); vegetable matter (plants, bark, roots etc.); and mineral substances (for instance, calcium and mineral salts). His *Materia Medica* sets out his observations and a detailed summary of the effects of the remedies, and constitutes a kind of dictionary of homeopathic medicines. Hahnemann's successors have expanded the *Materia Medica* by adding dilutions of human secretions and excretions, including pus and throat swabs, and more recently with chemical products, including pollutants and other toxins. Far from remaining fixed in its original concepts, homeopathy has continued to evolve over time. It is an adaptable therapy rather than a dogma. For instance, it was recently discovered that taking barbiturates over a long period could cause rheumatic problems, accompanied by pain and deformation of the shoulders and hands, to such an extent that the condition was described as 'gardenalic rheumatism' (from the name of one of the most common barbiturates). Thus, if confronted with rheumatism of this type, whatever the cause, the prescription of barbiturate dilutions (phenobarbitone) by a homeopathic doctor can bring significant relief.

**HOMEOPATHY AS SEEN BY THE FRENCH CARICATURIST, DAUMIER**

*'... Take a tiny grain of ... nothing ... divide it into 10 million molecules. Throw one of them ... in the river ... grind .... dilute this water with 20 parts of ordinary water and moisten the tongue with it every morning ...'*

### 'BLIND' TESTING

Hahnemann very quickly learned to take into account the constitution and predisposition of his human 'guinea pigs', in order to avoid confusing some of the signs with symptoms resulting directly from the experimentation. During his lifetime, trials were carried out on fit and healthy subjects in order to assess the effects of medicines (a process known as homeopathic proving), and also, on patients who were unaware of what was being tested on them and were thus 'blind'. This was to avoid any psychosomatic reactions. The pursuit of scientific discipline in order to test medicines was unknown at this time, but the technique, developed by Hahnemann and known as 'blind' testing, is still used nowadays to test the majority of modern medicines. Clinical researchers have improved research methods with the introduction of placebos. These are neutral products such as flavoured water or sugar pills used in place of a drug or remedy. Double blind experiments test the product on two identical groups, one taking the product to be tested and the other taking the placebo. Neither the subjects nor the doctors know which group they belong to. This technique was refined in the 20th century and is now used to test all drugs before they are put on the market. The 'blind' and 'double blind' techniques were actually discovered and perfected by homeopathic researchers, so it is rather

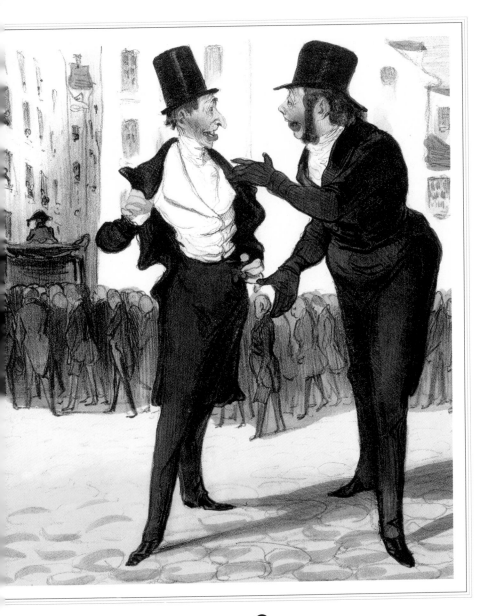

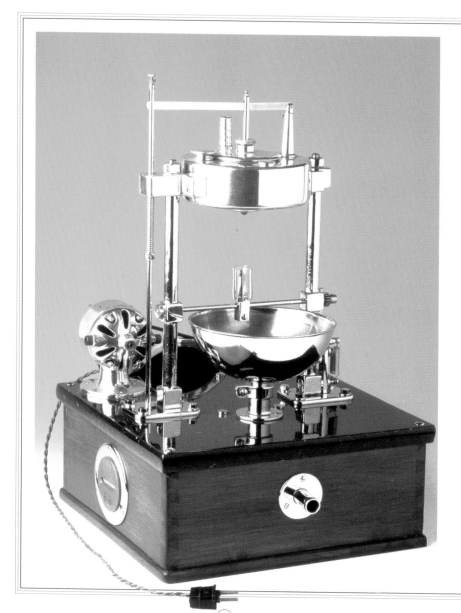

ironic to hear people say that homeopathy is nothing more than a placebo when, in fact, it was homeopathy that introduced this practice into modern pharmacological research.

## THE WORLD OF THE INFINITELY SMALL

The dilution process which Hahnemann invented enabled him to treat from the outset using minute doses, even though the science of his day was still unable to work them out or evaluate them precisely. The expression 'homeopathic dose' means 'almost nothing' and it is interesting to note that certain medical specialties, such as the study of allergies, have also come to use very small doses which, if not truly infinitesimal, are nonetheless minute.

The fact that homeopathic medicines contain so little of the active ingredient puts some people off and convinces them that this method cannot really work. 'You have to believe in homeopathy' or 'homeopathy is a placebo' are typical responses. But if that is the case, then how can we explain that this therapy works not only on humans, who can be influenced psychologically, but also on plants and animals? Take the example of chlorella, the small algae that make surface water green in hot countries and produce oxygen. If chlorella samples are put into a jar, their energy can be calculated exactly by analysing their oxygen output. If copper sulphate is added, they react immediately and their oxygen output decreases. They die if the dose is too high. Yet when a few drops of copper sulphate dilution are added to the jar, the chlorella start to produce oxygen again. These vegetable micro-organisms are thus 'sensitive' to what can be described as homeopathic treatment.

**GRINDING MACHINE**

*Non-soluble substances, ground in a mortar, are mixed with lactose until a powder is obtained which can be dissolved in a solvent.*

## HOMEOPATHY CAN BE USED TO TREAT ANIMALS

In 1796 Hahnemann wrote: 'If the laws of medicine which I acknowledge and proclaim are genuine, true and natural, they must apply to animals as well as people.' By the early 19th century, a Leipzig veterinary surgeon, Dr Lux, was already making homeopathic medicines which he administered to horses and cattle. A hundred and fifty years later, in northern France Dr Dehecq produced a homeopathic medicine, Wombyl (made up of *Actaea racemosa*, *Aletris farinosa* and *Caulophylum*), which enabled thousands of animals to give birth without difficulty. During the 1950s, at Lariboisière hospital in Paris, 2,000 mice were given large doses of oestrogen before being treated with homeopathic dilutions of this same hormone, with the result that the symptoms produced by the heavy dose of oestrogen decreased in a significant manner. In 1955, in Strasbourg, Professors Lapp and Wurmser gave rats, previously drugged with arsenic, a 7c dilution of this same poison. The treatment saved the rats lives. Several years ago, a species of oyster (Belon) was devastated by an unknown illness. A veterinary surgeon had the idea of making homeopathic dilutions from the sick oysters with which he then sprayed the spats (young oysters) resulting in the species being saved from extinction.

Veterinary medicine is thoroughly scientific and the homeopathic treatment of animals has existed for about one hundred and fifty years, a period corresponding to that of intensive farming. However, organic farming, which has emerged more recently, is especially sympathetic to homeopathic treatment of animals because the animal's bodies have not been weakened by the overuse of artificial foodstuffs or antibiotics. Homeopathic medicines do not produce side effects or toxic reactions and so offer the farmer healthier animals and, therefore, higher profits. In Britain, only a qualified veterinary surgeon is legally allowed to treat sick animals, but there are, however, a small number of homeopathic vets.

**VETERINARY HOMEOPATHY**

*According to government regulations, the milk of a sick cow treated with antibiotics is unusable for several weeks for health reasons, whilst it remains wholesome following homeopathic treatment.*

## THE DEVELOPMENT OF CLINICAL TRIALS

There have been numerous clinical trials of homeopathic medicine. Those using animals are particularly persuasive because animals respond well to the treatment but cannot be said to believe in it. This is difficult for some to accept as it is still not known precisely how homeopathy works, even though a significant number of trials have demonstrated its effectiveness. However, the distinction must be made between clinical studies, which evaluate a medicine's effectiveness by using people carrying the disease *in vivo*, and biological investigations, which study the effect of minimal doses of homeopathic medicines on living cells under laboratory conditions, *in vitro*. If the latter have not yet provided an answer which satisfies the whole of the scientific community, the first type of study clearly proves that homeopathic medicines do work.

Of the many successful experiments which have been carried out, one published in the scientific journal *The Lancet* by Dr David Reilly, of the Glasgow Homeopathic Hospital, demonstrates the effectiveness of homeopathy in the treatment of allergic rhinitis. The study focused on 158 patients of both sexes who, in the absence of any other treatment, received a dose twice daily of either 30 c pollen dilution, or a placebo. The symptoms decreased sharply and were statistically significant in the group treated by the homeopathic medicine.

Another study, carried out in Italy, set out to treat sixty patients suffering from migraines. Eight homeopathic remedies were used and while only 17 per cent of those given a placebo felt better, 93 per cent of those given homeopathic medicine experienced relief. Equally important

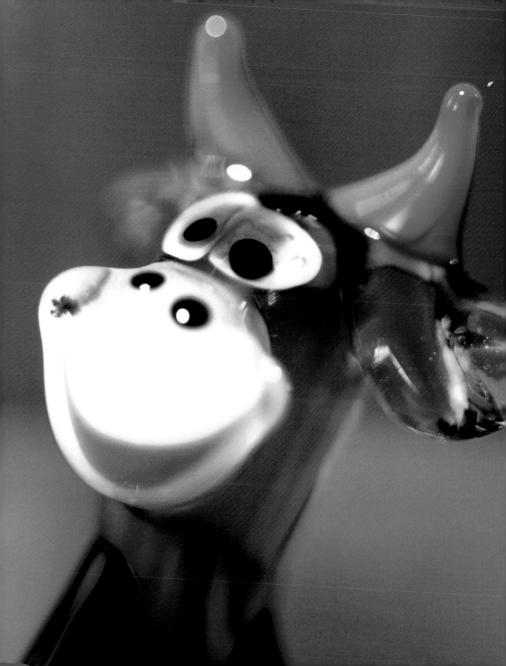

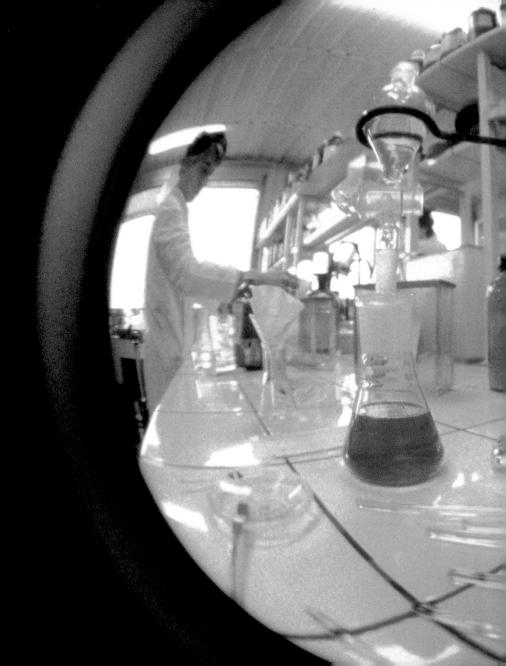

is the work that has been carried out in Nicaragua on the effect of homeopathy in the treatment of acute diarrhoea in children, and the work in Britain demonstrating the effectiveness of homeopathic medicines in the treatment of hay fever, rheumatoid arthritis and fibrositis.

Some studies, however, have produced negative results. On closer inspection, it is often construed that the experiments which failed to demonstrate the effectiveness of homeopathy were flawed because they did not correspond to the key principle of homeopathy – that it is an individualised treatment. The same remedy cannot be given to all patients suffering from a given illness, only to those whose pathology manifests itself in a similar way to a tested medicine. Nevertheless, homeopathy is, statistically speaking, an effective therapy. This is shown by a meta-analysis, which studies the overall statistical results of a hundred clinical trials. The three professors of medicine leading this investigation concluded that the overall results showed a positive trend, whatever the quality of the trials or the type of homeopathic prescription used.

## HOMEOPATHY IN LABORATORY TESTS

Homeopathic research can also be of interest to the work carried out in other scientific or medical spheres. One of the most well known, and widely publicised works of this nature was carried out by a French scientist, Jacques Benveniste. At the end of the 1980s, Benveniste was in charge of a unit of the French National Institute of Medical Research (INSERM). Although not a homeopath himself, he was responsible for an investigation focusing on the effect of infinitesimal dilutions of histamine on immune cells. In view of the results obtained, he offered an explanation, which was published in the English scientific journal, *Nature*. In his opinion, the effectiveness of homeopathic dilutions is to be found in the structure of water itself, which is capable of retaining the 'memory' of the active molecules that have passed through it. It wasn't long before some members of the scientific community reacted against his hypothesis, considering it to be a hoax. The debate about the 'memory of water' received extensive coverage both in the scientific and also the popular press. Some laboratories subsequently undertook the same experiments and obtained identical results to Benveniste. Others maintained that the experiments could not be reproduced, whilst some tried to prove that he had cheated. To this day, even if Jacques Benveniste and his collaborators have not succeeded in getting the scientific community to admit they were right, no one has been able to prove them wrong.

**HOMEOPATHIC RESEARCH**

*Research into homeopathy is very active in some countries with large investments from government and pharmaceutical companies, but in Britain, homeopathic research is mostly charitably funded.*

In the mid-1980s, Professor Madeleine Bastide, of the immunology laboratory of Montpellier University pharmacology faculty, studied the action of infinitesimal hormone doses on the immune cells. This work demonstrated that a product, even when diluted to the extreme, retains a biological action. Moreover, this action differs according to the dilution, the less of the initial product that remains in the solution that is used, the greater its action. More recently, at the University of Bordeaux haematology unit, the effects of aspirin dilutions on blood coagulation were studied. It was proved that an aspirin dilution possesses the opposite action to aspirin administered by weight, in this case actually producing coagulation. Other experiments have demonstrated the action of *Apis mellifica* on the modulation of certain immune cells (basophils), and that of *Silica* on the reaction of the macrophagic cells, whose function is to eliminate any undesirable micro-organism which enters the body.

## HOW DOES IT WORK?

Many things remain to be discovered to enable an explanation of the effectiveness of homeopathy which will be acceptable to the scientific community. For the moment, some doctors are attempting to bridge the gap, for example, Dr Michel Conan Mériadec, President of the French School of Homeopathy who describes Hahnemann's process as follows: 'The principle of similarity is the result of a process which can be described as experimental, since it was based on an observation, giving rise to a hypothesis, which was confirmed by experimentation. This accords with scientific methodology which can be said to proceed as follows:

1. The observation: the statement that there is an analogy of symptoms between a natural illness and the illness medicinally induced by the homeopathic remedy which is used to treat this illness empirically.

2. The hypothesis: "like treats like", the medicine treats the illness because it causes a similar illness in a healthy person.

3. The proof is shown in two ways: via a pathogenic study of the medicines which involves using substances to induce illness; and through therapeutic testing, which demonstrates that minute doses of the same medicines can provide a cure, so like does treat like.'

One of the hypotheses most recently put forward to explain the way homeopathy works is based on the idea that there is an analogy between the structure of the homeopathic medicine and the deficiency in the physiology of the body which gives rise to an illness. The medicine therefore acts like a key, which is able to unlock the dysfunctional system.

**THE MEMORY OF WATER**

*During successive dilutions, water has been shown to retain the trace of the substance which has passed through it, to the extent that it continues to deliver a therapeutic message.*

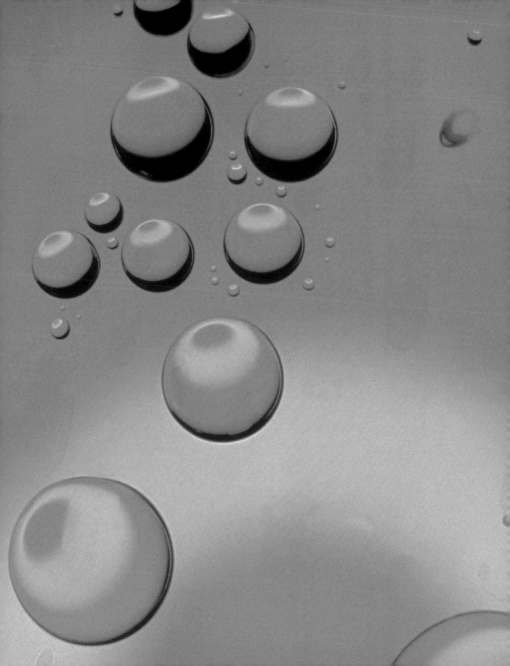

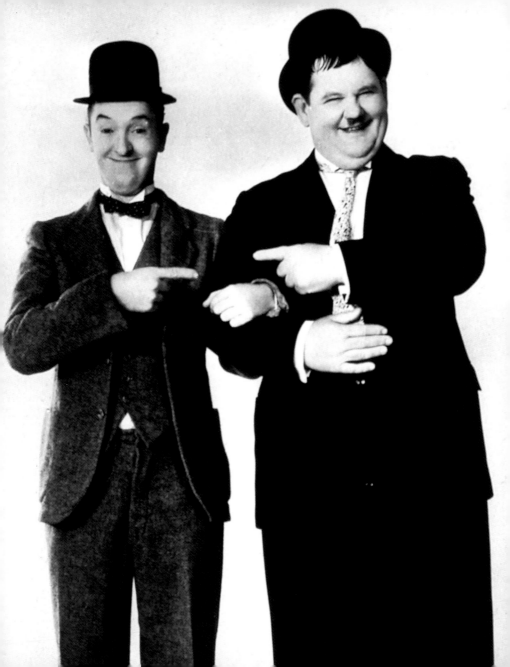

## WHAT REMAINS OF HAHNEMANN'S DISCOVERIES?

As well as the principle of similarity and the process of homeopathic dilutions, the notion of constitution is one of Hahnemann's basic principles. This is defined as the inherited and acquired physical, emotional and intellectual make-up of an individual. Hahnemann suggested that each constitutional type had a particular susceptibility to illness which might be invoked as a result of environmental or individual stresses which could be mental, emotional or physical. Hahnemann also formed a theory of chronic illnesses which he called miasms. A miasm was the result of an inherited predisposition to a particular kind of illness which meant that the patients did not respond to homeopathic medicines or suffered frequent relapses. Susceptibility and diathesis make up the individual's medicinal picture, on the basis of observation, and to the homeopathic doctor they constitute an excellent way of establishing an individual's basic state of health and future prognosis.

**HOMEOPATHY AND CONSTITUTION**

*The homeopath adapts his prescription to the patient's constitution, build, psychological profile and medical history. Laurel and Hardy would be treated differently if suffering from the same illness.*

Before reaching such a refined level of theory, the therapy perfected by Samuel Hahnemann went through numerous stages of development, before it became firmly established throughout the world. In 1832, a French doctor, Dr Sébastien Des Guidi (1785–1864) became interested in this innovation and published a *Letter to French doctors about homeopathy* in order to spread information about homeopathy throughout the medical world. Two years later, in 1834, Georg Jahr, Hahnemann's secretary and friend, settled in Paris, where he published a manual to facilitate the study and use of homeopathic medicines. France thus became one of the first countries to be closely involved in homeopathy and was also home to the world's first homeopathic pharmaceutical laboratory. Clemens Maria von Boenninghausen, another of Hahnemann's relatives, compiled the first *Homeopathic Repertory* in 1832. That same year, the Homeopathic Society of Paris was founded, bringing together a growing number of practitioners. Homeopathy would subsequently be talked about at every possible opportunity. This was particularly the case during the cholera epidemics that affected the whole of Europe during the middle of the 19th century when homeopathic doctors obtained results where classical medicine had previously failed.

## THE SPREAD OF A NEW THERAPY

Since Hahnemann's death, and in keeping with his wishes, homeopathy has spread throughout Europe and the rest of the world driven by the work of enthusiastic and motivated doctors. In Italy the important figures were Horatis (1770–1850) and Romani (1788–1853); in Spain Iriarte,

Querol, Nunez y Pernia (1805–1879) and Metges (1821–1900); in Portugal, around 1848, Padstor and D'Alcantara; in Great Britain Quin (1789–1878), Hughes (1836–1902) and Clarke (1853–1931); in Ireland Luther; and in 1826, Wallenberg, in Sweden. Homeopathy was promoted by Marenzeller (1765–1854) in Austria, de Moor (1787–1845) in Belgium, Schonfeld, in 1834, in Holland, Dufresne, the same year in Switzerland, and in Russia from 1823, with Adam and Trisnius, Hahnemann's nephew, who also circulated his principles in Poland and Eastern Europe. During the 1830s, Benoît Mure, a young man from Lyons who was successfully treated with homeopathy, embarked on a crusade to spread this revolutionary medicine through Malta, Sicily and Brazil, and later Egypt. His great achievement was the opening, in 1843, of the Institute of Homeopathy in Brazil.

Homeopathy was practised in India after 1841 following the creation of a faculty in Bengal. Gandhi very quickly declared himself in favour of homeopathy which he described as 'ecological and economical', making it accessible to everyone, including the poorest. In India, today, there are over 100,000 homeopathic doctors, while in France there are an estimated 5,000 doctors using homeopathy. In Britain there are around 2,000 homeopaths, divided equally between lay homeopaths and medically qualified homeopathic doctors.

In Britain, homeopathy was espoused by the work of Frederick Foster Hervey Quin, who, in 1831, was cured of cholera by *camphor* and thereafter was so convinced of the efficacy of the therapy that he founded his own practice in London in 1832 and later established the first homeopathic hospital in London in 1849. Quin treated many famous people, including the writers Dickens and Thackeray. In the latter part of the century homeopathic hospitals were established in Bristol, Liverpool, Glasgow and Tunbridge Wells, and in 1948, when the National Health Service was established, homeopathy was included as a viable form of treatment. The British Royal Family are staunch supporters and by the end of the 20th century, homeopathy had become widely available in Britain. In addition to its availability through the National Health Service, homeopathy has played a central role in the general growth of interest in complementary medicine. Interest in homeopathy also spread to Australia and New Zealand where it is now widely available.

**EXPANSION IN THE 19TH CENTURY**

*Thanks to the conviction of some enthusiasts, homeopathy spread from Germany throughout the whole of Europe and the rest of the world. Doctors like Quin in Britain, Kent in America, Hering in Germany and Des Guidi in France passionately embraced the new therapy.*

In the United States, the American Institute of Homeopathy was founded in 1844, thanks to Constantin Hering (1800–1880). He was succeeded by other doctors, including Farrington, Allen and Nash. A very special mention must be reserved for the American homeopath, James Tyler Kent (1849–1916), who developed the theory of constitutional types – people of a similar

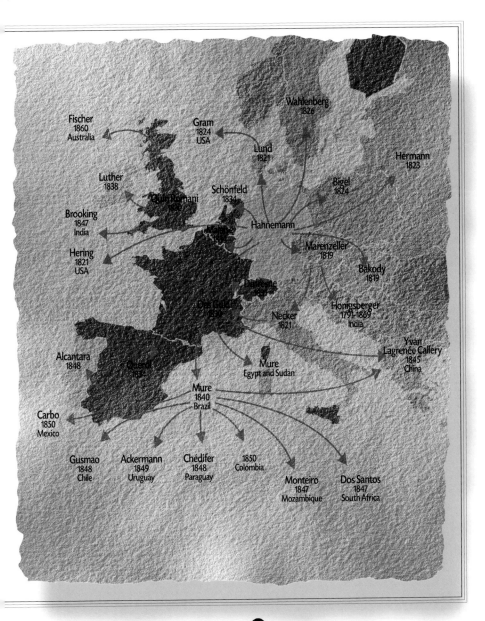

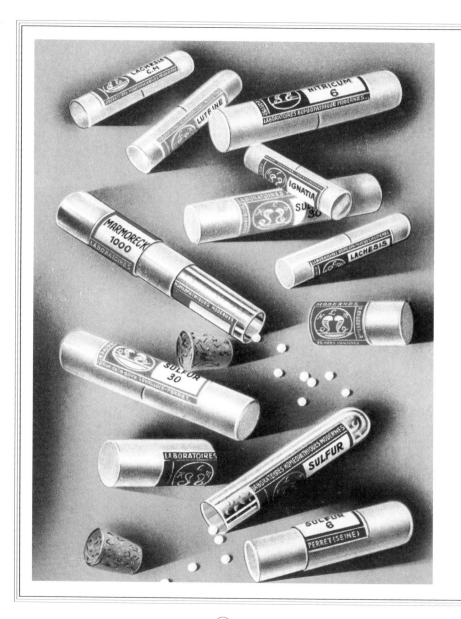

emotional make-up who tend to develop the same diseases and therefore are specifically suited to some remedies. For instance, *Natrum mur* types are said to be pear-shaped with dark complexions, of a reserved and fastidious nature, salt craving and constipated. Kent's major works are his *Repertory*, often re-published and sometimes thought of as a 'homeopathic bible', his *Materia Medica* and his *Philosophy*. Kent developed the practice of prescribing remedies in high potencies which led to a split amongst American homeopaths as to the correct level of dosage. The initiative of these men helped the spread of homeopathy to Canada, particularly Quebec.

In Latin America, other institutes opened in addition to the one in Brazil: in Chile in 1848 by Gusmao; in Paraguay in 1848 by Chedifer; in Uruguay in 1849 by Ackerman; in Mexico in 1850 by Cormellos and Carbo; and in Argentina in 1934 by Paschero. On the African continent, Dos Santos introduced homeopathy to South Africa in 1846 and Montero introduced it to Mozambique in 1847.

**PACKAGING**

*In France, until the 1960s, granules and globules, the most common homeopathic forms, were sold in glass containers, themselves enclosed in an aluminium tube fastened by a cork.*

After homeopathy became established in France, homeopathic training began, primarily at the Saint-Jacques hospital in Paris, which was founded in 1870 and still exists. In 1931 it officially became the Paris School of Homeopathy. The French Homeopathic Society was formed in 1889. In modern France, only medically qualified doctors, dentists, midwives and veterinarians may practise homeopathy. Training takes place at one of seven universities, or at schools of medicine or at one of the private schools run by manufacturers of homeopathic medicine. In February 1998, homeopathy was recognised as a therapy by the French National Medical Authority, which officially requested its serious scientific evaluation as well as its introduction into the medical curriculum.

## THE AVAILABILITY OF HOMEOPATHIC MEDICINES

At the start of the 21st century, homeopathy is available more or less all over the world. While doctors, chemists and veterinary surgeons work in an individual capacity, some pharmaceutical laboratories also help with the spread and development of this therapy in new countries. Hahnemann and his immediate successors produced the dilutions and medicines themselves. Few modern homeopaths produce their own remedies. Instead, manufacturing methods range from small pharmacies producing remedies by hand to large companies with their own pharmaceutical laboratories using strictly controlled procedures. Homeopathic medicines are freely available in chemists' shops in Britain as well as in health food stores, by mail order and through the Internet. They are also supplied directly by homeopaths and homeopathic hospitals following consultations. The sale of homeopathic medicines in British pharmacies is increasing by an estimated 15–20 per cent per year while GP referrals to the NHS homeopathic hospitals are also rising steadily. A survey carried out by the *British Medical Journal (BMJ)* in 1994 showed that 80 per cent of the newly qualified doctors who were interviewed wished to train in homeopathy or another complementary therapy.

Homeopathic medicines are less expensive than conventional drugs and it seems that patients who use homeopathy are ill less often. The cost of homeopathic medicine makes it particularly suited to the problems of developing countries and no doubt, in part, explains its success in India where there are an estimated 100,000 homeopathic practitioners. In 1994, a random clinical trial held in Nicaragua on the treatment of childhood diarrhoea with homeopathic medicine, showed a definite reduction in the severity and duration of the attack for those children given homeopathic treatment. Homeopathy is widespread in South America as well as parts of Africa and south east Asia. The World Health Organisation has said: 'Homeopathic treatment seems well suited for use in rural areas where the infrastructure, equipment and drugs needed for conventional medicine cannot be provided.'

### HOMEOPATHY IS A TYPE OF MEDICINE WHICH RESPECTS THE INDIVIDUAL

Scientific knowledge continues to make great advances but, as it does so, it demonstrates with each new discovery the immeasurable territory that remains uncharted. However, ignoring this obvious fact, there are many who place on orthodox medicine a responsibility that it is unable to fulfill: that it must cure everything immediately. For example, during the 1970s, new medicines were developed to treat high blood pressure. These medicines were described as revolutionary but turned out to be effective for some patients only.

We all react differently to pain and illness, and homeopathy takes account of this. By considering the person who is suffering and not just the illness, it simultaneously takes into account the symptoms, the patient's constitution and even his psychological and emotional reactions. In a case such as high blood pressure, it can thus confront both the causes and effects of the condition. It can also be combined with allopathic treatments in two ways: firstly, the homeopathic interpretation of the patient's constitution enables the practitioner to choose, from the array of remedies at his disposal, the one which is best suited to the individual patient; secondly, homeopathic treatment used in conjunction with allopathic drugs enables a reduction in drug dosages and unwanted side effects.

**GRANULES**

*There are many types of packaging for homeopathic medicines. Granules, for example, are often dispensed in tubes, equipped with dosage caps which, when pushed downwards, release the required number of granules.*

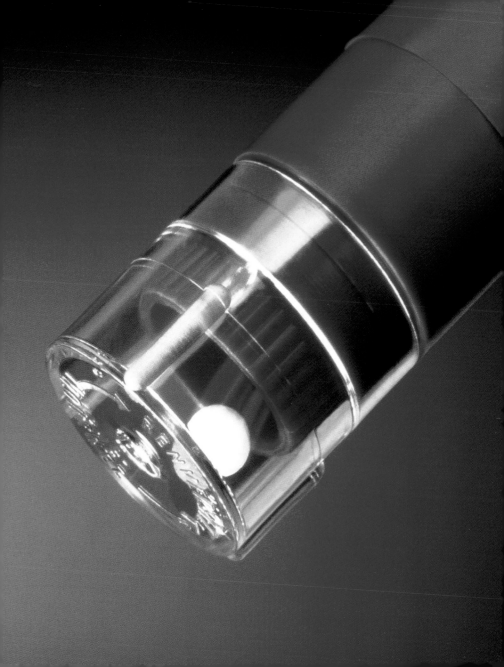

Doctors in Britain are increasingly interested in studying homeopathy and surveys have shown that over two-thirds of doctors would like to be able to refer their patients for homeopathic or other complementary medicine.

## HOMEOPATHY IS THE THERAPY OF THE FUTURE

Homeopathy can be considered a therapy of the future in more ways than one. The more acute the illness, the quicker it is cured by homeopathy. In the case of chronic illnesses, it enables a reduction in the use of orthodox, and sometimes toxic, medicines and hence their side effects. It is also a fundamentally ecological practice as it does not harm the patient or the environment. The environment is increasingly polluted by waste from modern medicines such as antibiotics. These accumulate in human or animal waste and also find their way into the food chain through routine use among farm animals. Homeopathic medicines are also acceptable to those concerned with animal welfare since they are produced without the need for animal experimentation.

The way homeopathy works is still not fully understood, but its use is growing rapidly, and as scientific trials multiply and confirm its efficacy, so science comes nearer to finding the answer. However, even when the answer is found, there remains the huge task of challenging the way medicine is practised. Let's hope that homeopathy has an influence on the understanding and perception of the patient as a holistic being.

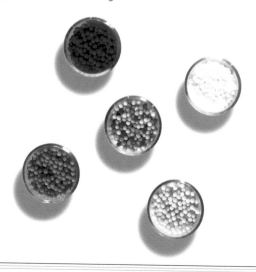

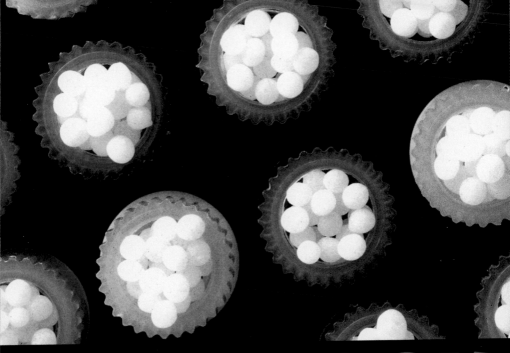

# LOOK

FROM THE PLANT TO THE MOTHER TINCTURE, THE MEDICINE IS
FINALLY READY. MANUFACTURING HOMEOPATHIC REMEDIES THE MODERN
WAY, FAR REMOVED FROM HAHNEMANN'S INITIAL EXPERIMENTS.
IMAGES FROM A HOMEOPATHIC LABORATORY.

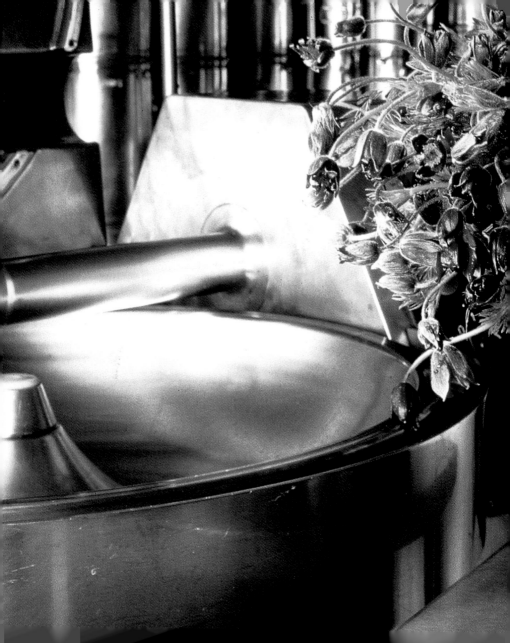

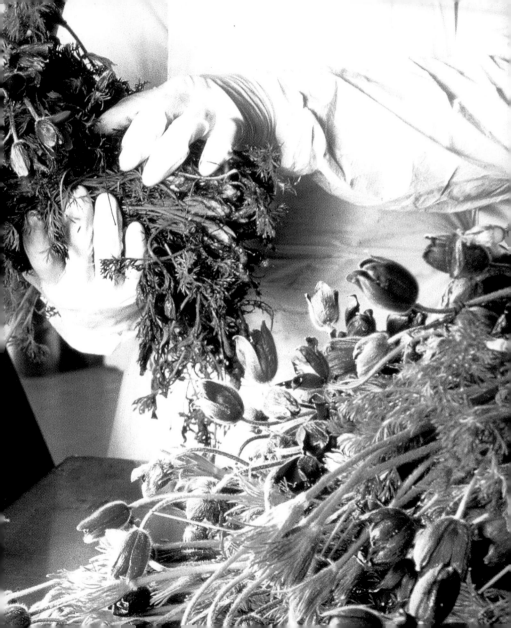

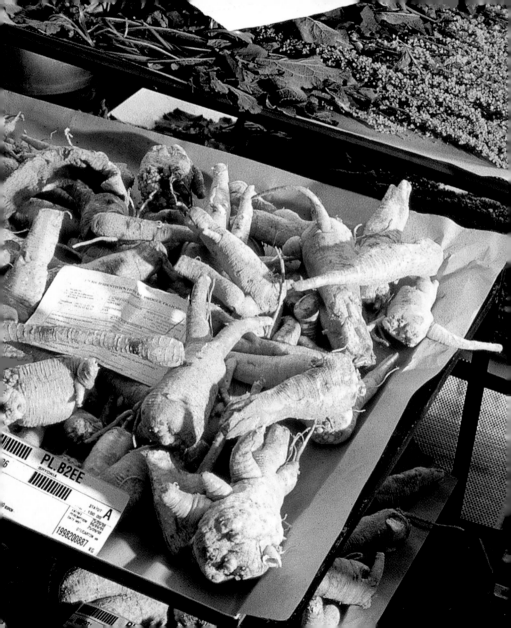

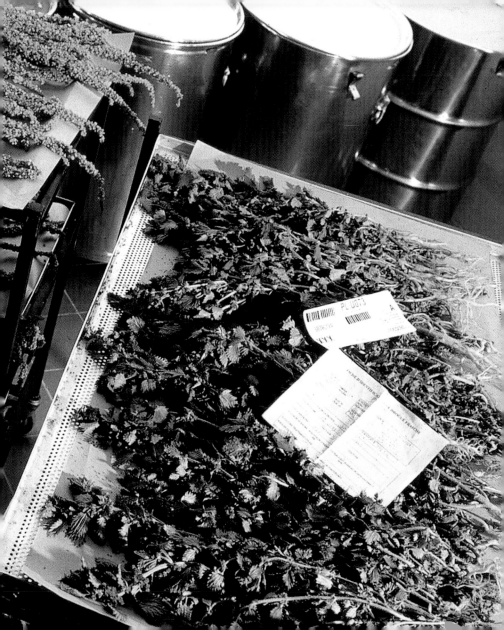

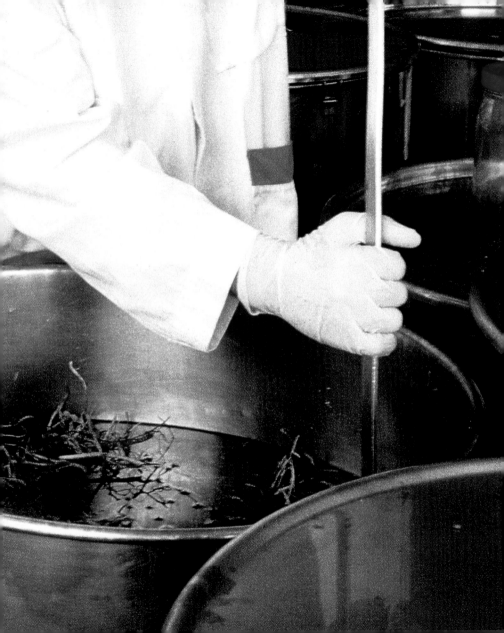

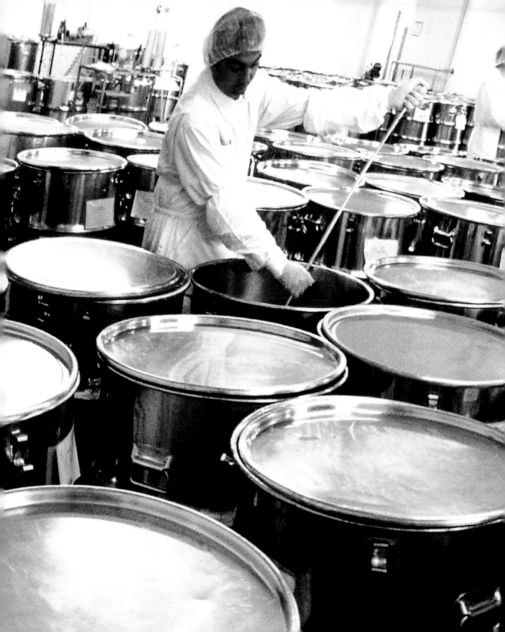

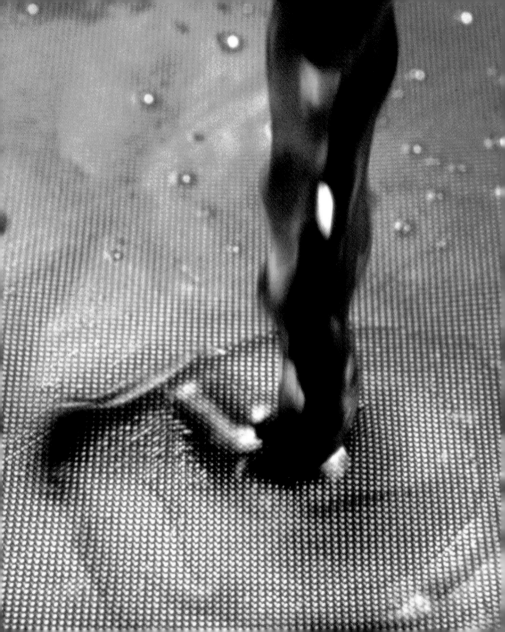

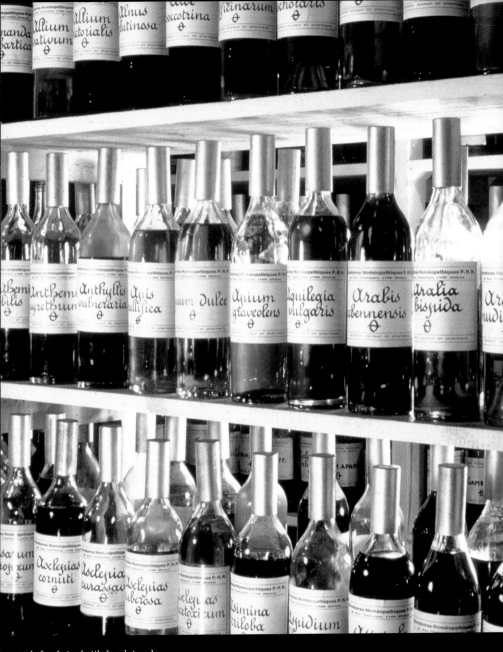

*... before being bottled and stored.*

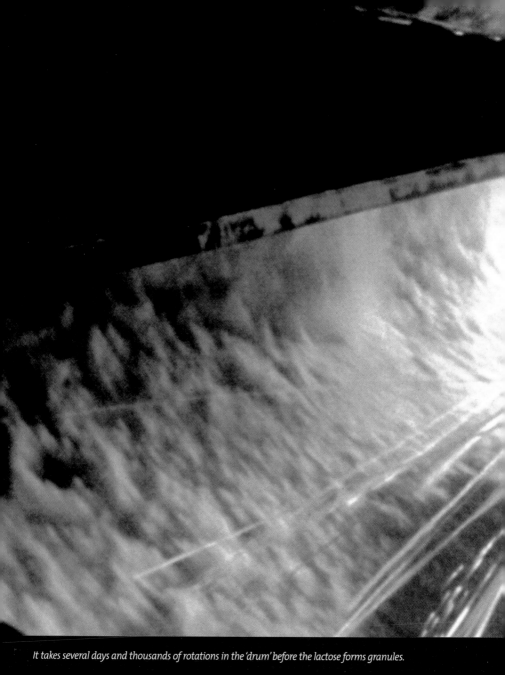

*It takes several days and thousands of rotations in the 'drum' before the lactose forms granules.*

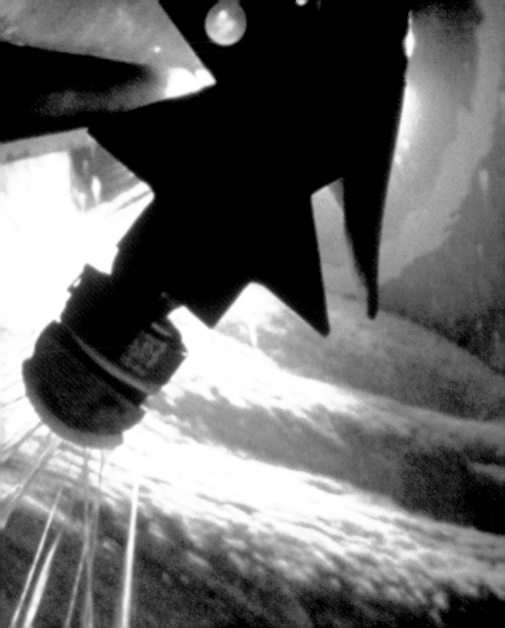

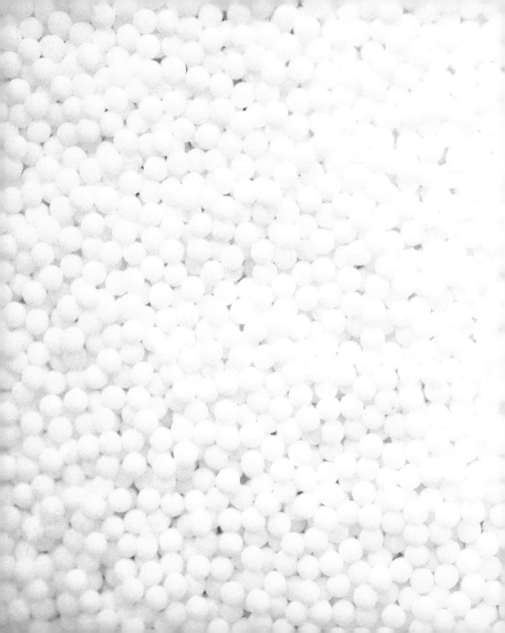

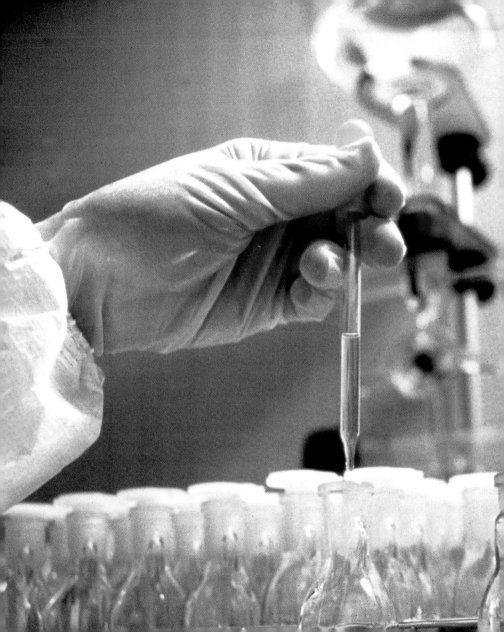

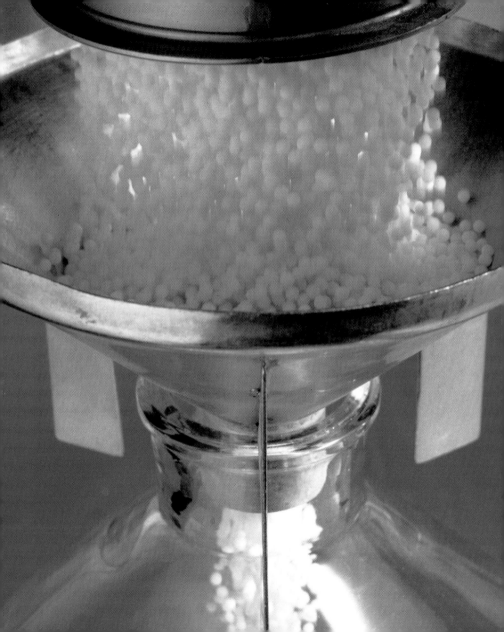

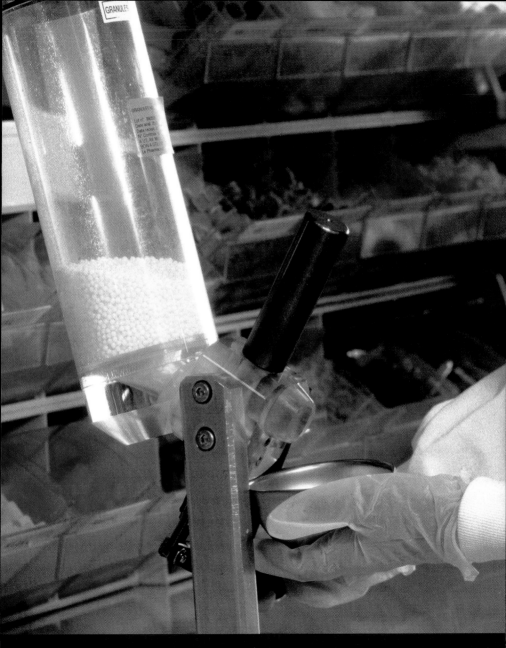

*Korsakov's dilutions are more common in English-speaking countries.*

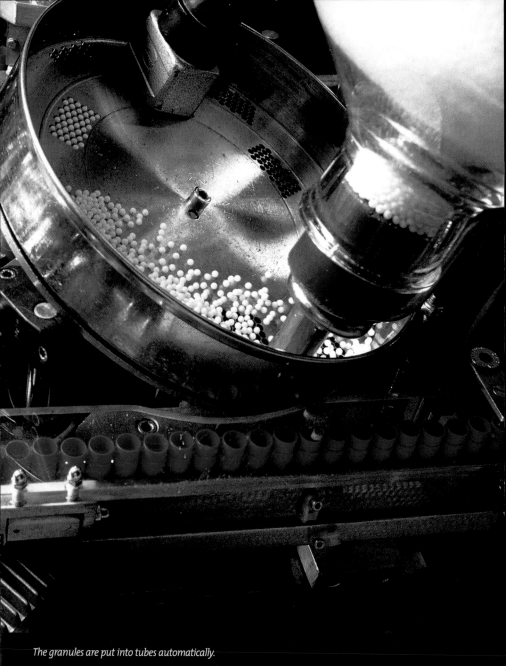
The granules are put into tubes automatically.

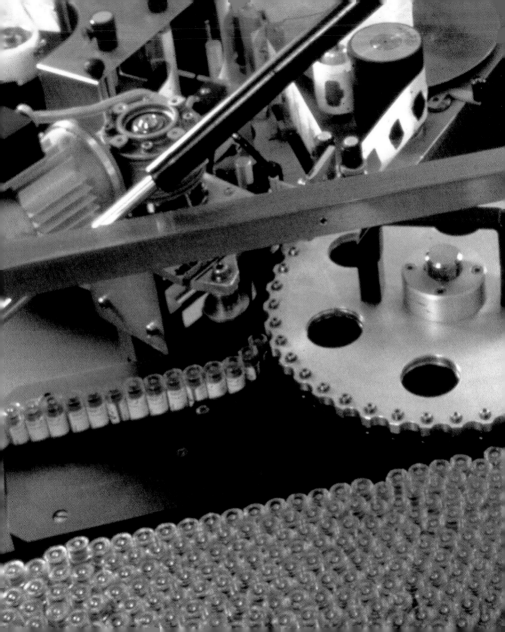

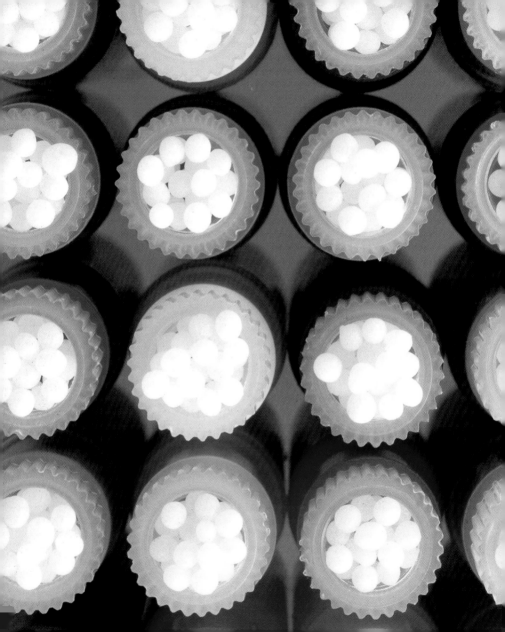

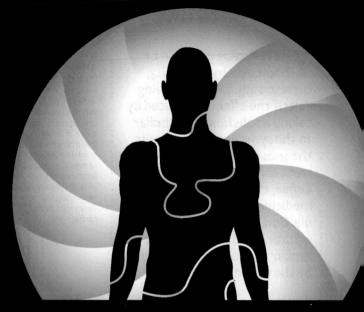

# IN PRACTICE

WHAT DOES 'LIKE TREATS LIKE' MEAN? HOW ARE POTENCIES MEASURED?
WHAT SHOULD YOU EXPECT FROM A HOMEOPATHIC CONSULTATION?
HOW DOES HOMEOPATHY FIT IN WITH CONVENTIONAL MEDICINE?
CAN YOU USE IT TO TREAT CHILDREN, THE ELDERLY AND EVEN PETS?
DO YOU NEED A DOCTOR'S PRESCRIPTION?

# Like treats like

**T**he founding principle of homeopathy, similarity, corresponds to the following rule: if the effects produced by taking a substance are similar to the symptoms of an illness, the substance in question can treat the illness. For example, *Coffea*, the homeopathic medicine based on coffee dilution, treats shaking, agitation and insomnia, effects similar to those experienced by the coffee drinker.

### Here are three examples
Each example pairs a homeopathic remedy with the illnesses or constitutional types for which it is recommended.

### Nux vomica and the quick-tempered, hyperactive individual

Impulsive, impatient, restless, hyperactive, periods of exhaustion and depression due to an excess of nervous energy; violent temper, unable to tolerate the least contradiction; vomiting, flatulence, constipation, piles; spasms, cramps, neuralgia, numbness; sleepy after meals; cardiac pains, palpitations, high blood pressure; sneezing, cold symptoms; cough, asthma; insomnia; over-sensitivity to odours; symptoms aggravated by anger, stimulants, cold dry weather; symptoms improved by sleep (all night or short nap) and warmth.

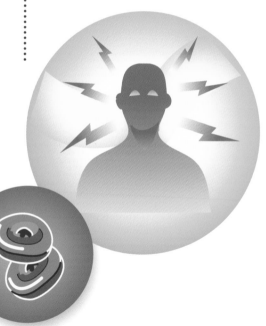

## Arsenicum album and the miser

Alternates between agitation and depression, or between internal and external symptoms (such as diarrhoea and eczema); very pronounced nervousness; body odour; anxiety; general weakness; burning pains (improved by warmth); thirst for small quantities of cold water; deformed extremities (claw-like hands); fear of failure; symptoms aggravated by cold and between 1 and 3 am; symptoms clearly improved by warmth.

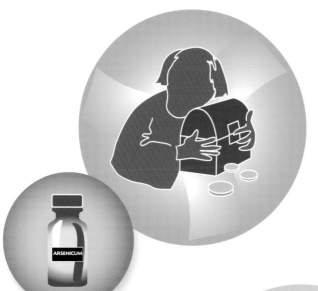

## Sepia and the sad, depressed woman

Sad, irritable and seeks solitude; weak joints; lumbar pain; venous congestion and irregular periods; cystitis; constipation; feeling of heaviness in the abdomen, lumps in the throat or stomach; craving for vinegar (or foods such as gherkins) and aversion to milk; various discharges; symptoms aggravated by consolation, cold or stale air and standing upright; symptoms improved by recreational activity and vigorous physical exercise such as tennis or jogging.

# Constitution and identifying constitutional types

**M**ost people have their strengths and weaknesses. One person will be susceptible to headaches, while another will have a weakness in the digestive system. In homeopathy the goal is to consider the whole situation of which the ailment or weakness is a part. To do this, homeopaths try to identify the constitutional type of the patient, although a person will never correspond completely to a single constitutional type. However, they represent a way of understanding the subject's sensibilities and responses.

## A recent notion

Although the idea of constitutional types has existed since the time of Hippocrates, it was not until the 20th century that this theory was revived by numerous medical practitioners, particularly within complementary medicine.

## The constitution

The homeopath has two methods at his disposal to help him work out the patient's constitution: the constitutional types, which clarify the patient's responses, and diathesis, which pinpoints weaknesses.

## The normative

Certain subjects – normatives – do not fall within any of the major constitutional types. Psychologically, they are very cerebral and enjoy life. They consume everything hungrily – information as well as food – which makes them untidy, disorganised and prone to constipation. Their base medicine is *Sulphur*.

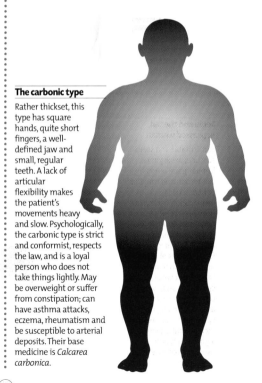

### The carbonic type

Rather thickset, this type has square hands, quite short fingers, a well-defined jaw and small, regular teeth. A lack of articular flexibility makes the patient's movements heavy and slow. Psychologically, the carbonic type is strict and conformist, respects the law, and is a loyal person who does not take things lightly. May be overweight or suffer from constipation; can have asthma attacks, eczema, rheumatism and be susceptible to arterial deposits. Their base medicine is *Calcarea carbonica*.

## The fluoric type

The silhouette is irregular and asymmetrical, like the teeth. This type has a gangling walk and great articular flexibility which gives a catlike appearance. Emotional and original in nature, the fluoric type likes novelty and has no fear of controversy. There may be a tendency to bone and ligament troubles as well as skin problems. Their base medicine is *Calcarea fluorica*.

## The phosphoric type

Tall, slim and slender, with elegant movements, this type has long, straight hands and an upper jaw which often juts out in relation to the lower. This person is emotional and easily excited, but just as easily deflated. Although rather refined with a love of beautiful things, they are also prone to fatigue with low resistance to infections, particularly of the ear, nose and throat. Their base medicine is *Calcarea phosphorica*.

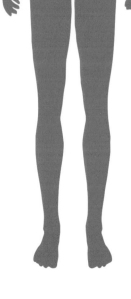

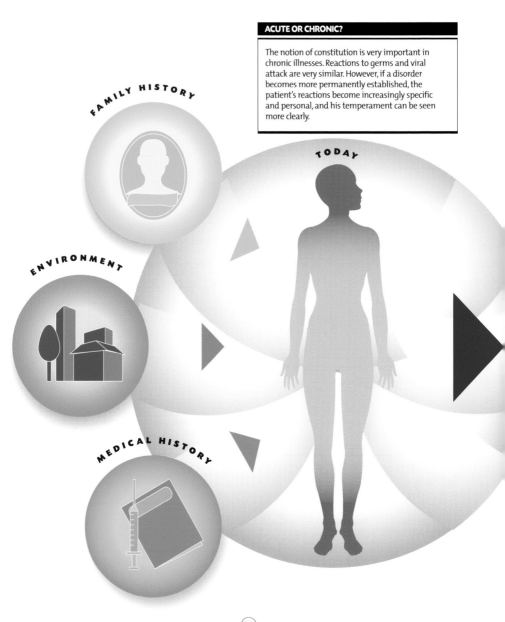

**ACUTE OR CHRONIC?**

The notion of constitution is very important in chronic illnesses. Reactions to germs and viral attack are very similar. However, if a disorder becomes more permanently established, the patient's reactions become increasingly specific and personal, and his temperament can be seen more clearly.

FAMILY HISTORY

ENVIRONMENT

MEDICAL HISTORY

TODAY

# Temperament and diathesis

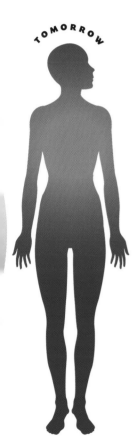

TOMORROW

The individual's diathesis is the sum of all the elements that characterise him or her at a given point in life: family background, medical history, living conditions, material and psychological environment. There are four types of diathesis: syphilitic, sycotic, tuberculinic and psoric. Each has its own way of reacting to illness. By carefully working out a patient's temperament – including tendencies, reactions and weaknesses – the homeopathic doctor can prescribe accurately and efficiently.

### Syphilitic

Psychologically unstable; inflammation can lead to lesions (from ulceration to sclerosis); deformations of the bones (exostosis) and ligaments (viscous; growth disorders); symptoms are worse during the night.

### Sycotic

Symptoms appear following infection (viral or bacteriological) or long-term chemical treatment (tablets); latent depression; water retention (oedemas, cellulite); sensitivity to humidity; chronic irritation of the mucous membranes; prone to cysts, verrucas and polyps.

### Tuberculinic

Psychological and sensory hypersensitivity; eating disorders (anorexia/bulimia, crash diets) which can upset growth; weight loss despite a healthy appetite; throat infections, bronchitis, digestive disorders linked to cold weather; chronic inflammation of the respiratory tracts (nose, throat and bronchial tubes); venous disorders of the circulation.

### Psoric

Symptoms appear after the withdrawal of treatment (a cold suddenly dries up, eczema dries out too quickly); alternates between pathological symptoms (asthma/ hives, digestive disorders/ rheumatism); alternates between improvements and relapses; periodical symptoms (seasonal or annual); thermo-regulatory disorders (too hot, too cold); circulatory disorders; abnormalities in appetite which might be associated with digestive disorders; prone to parasitosis (diseases caused by parasite infestations).

# The manufacture of homeopathic medicines

**H**omeopathy often uses products of an animal, vegetable, mineral or chemical origin which, in their natural state, can be dangerous. So, to eliminate any risk of poisoning, each base substance is diluted several times and processed to produce a medicine containing infinitesimal doses.

**Where do the raw materials come from?**

Homeopathy uses approximately 3,500 substances, including insects, animal venoms, mineral extracts, vegetable toxins and chemical molecules. These are subject to very strict controls, including checks for radioactive pollution, pesticides and fertilisers in order to guarantee their absolute purity. The wild plants are taken from nature and the domestic plants are produced by organic farming. The animal samples are taken by veterinary surgeons.

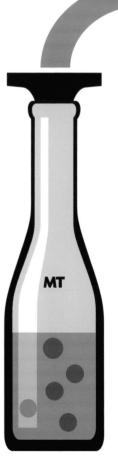

**THE MOTHER TINCTURE**

For a plant or a whole animal (such as the bee), the base substance is first steeped in a solvent (alcohol and water) for 21 days. A dried mineral, chemical or animal substance (such as dried venom) is ground before being mixed with the solvent. In both cases, the mixture is pressed and filtered, to produce the mother tincture.

MT

## Hahnemann's dilutions

Hahnemann's centesimal scale uses dilutions of 1 in 100. One drop of mother tincture is added to 99 drops of alcohol, then shaken vigorously: this is known as potentisation.

The result is a dilution of 1 c, that is a concentration of 1:100. Then mix one drop of this first dilution with 99 drops of alcohol; potentise to obtain a dilution of 2 c, that is a concentration of 1:10,000.

Mix one drop of this second dilution with 99 drops of alcohol; potentise to obtain a dilution of 3 c, that is a concentration of 1:1,000,000; and so on. This method of dilution

is one way of making homeopathic medicine. Hahnemann's dilutions are the most commonly used in Britain, but Korsakov's dilutions are also available (see page 74).

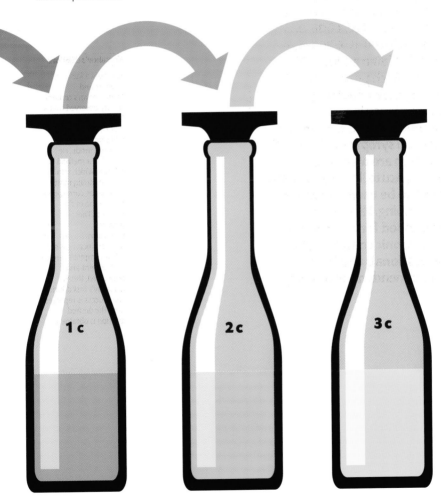

1 c

2 c

3 c

# The potencies

It is customary to refer to low (6 to 12 c), medium (30 c) or high potencies. High potencies are referred to as 200:1 m (diluted 1,000 times), 50 m (diluted 50,000 times) and CM (diluted 100,000 times). Each potency has its own sphere of activity. Low potency is more commonly used for specific physical symptoms; low and medium are often used during acute illnesses but 30 c can also be used for chronic prescribing. High potency is prescribed for constitutional and chronic conditions by professionals and is not recommended for self help.

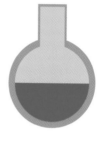

**Korsakov's dilutions**

Korsakov, a Russian chemist and Hahnemann's contemporary, observed that a bottle which has previously been emptied still contains liquid residues inside. He invented a method of dilution which retains the remaining matter, in two stages, corresponding to 1:100 of the contents. These dilutions are made by filling a bottle with the mother tincture, which is then emptied, refilled with solvent and potentised; this is Korsakov's first dilution. The process is repeated until the desired dilution is obtained.

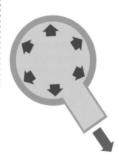

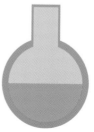

New observation techniques have revealed differences in the composition of dilutions produced by each method. When a bottle is filled with the diluted mixture to prepare a Korsakov dilution, the molecules have a greater tendency to distribute themselves towards the sides of the bottle. The amount of the active element contained in the dilutions of Hahnemann and Korsakov is thus not exactly the same.

The dilutions of Hahnemann and Korsakov each act in a different way, particularly where high potencies are concerned. The high potencies of Korsakov's dilution have a milder, more subtle action, and are more effective psychologically. Since Korsakov's dilutions are always made in the same bottle, the final product contains a mixture of all the successive dilutions. So, in some cases, giving a patient the same medicine diluted to different degrees can change or increase the effect.

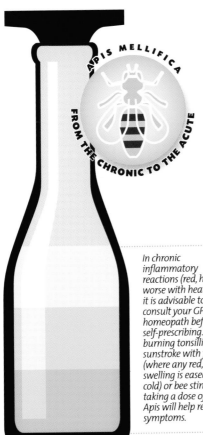

In chronic inflammatory reactions (red, hot, worse with heat) it is advisable to consult your GP or homeopath before self-prescribing. For burning tonsillitis, sunstroke with fever (where any red, hot swelling is eased by cold) or bee stings, taking a dose of Apis will help relieve symptoms.

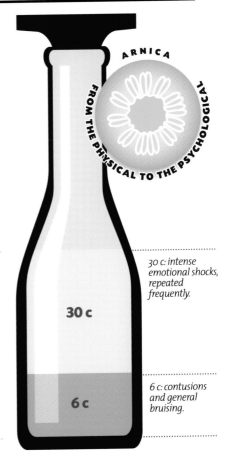

30 c: intense emotional shocks, repeated frequently.

6 c: contusions and general bruising.

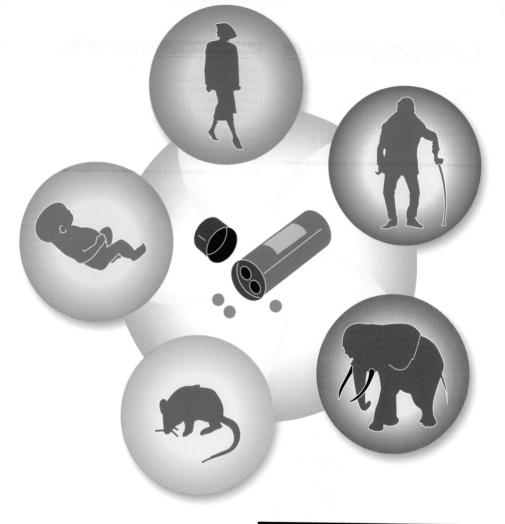

**PILLS OR COARSE GRANULES AND LMs**

Pills (soft and hard), coarse granules and LMs (liquid preparations) are the most common way to take homeopathic medicine. Low potency doses and LMs allow the medicine to be repeated at regular intervals until the body reacts. The LM scale is based on a dilution at a ratio of 1 in 50,000. Usually dispensed in drops, it is not very commonly used.

# Actions and reactions

The same quantity of granules can be used to treat an elephant or a mouse, and an infant or an elderly person, since there is no real link between the amount of product taken and its effectiveness. It is pointless to increase the dosage, as taking twice as much will not speed up the effect.

### To treat an acute illness
The more acute and recent the illness, the quicker the action of the homeopathy. The treatment can be stopped as soon as the symptoms subside or stop, unlike antibiotics, which must be taken for a certain period of time. Homeopathy can be likened to a lumberjack felling a tree; if he fells it when it is young he can simply cut the trunk but, if he waits too long, he must first remove many of the branches before the whole tree can be felled.

### To treat a chronic illness
In chronic illness, prolonged treatments may be necessary, but may have no obvious immediate effect. It is possible to gradually space out the doses of homeopathic medicine and then take them again more frequently if the symptoms reappear. Here, the homeopathic action can be compared to that of a fertiliser: if the ground is enriched in winter, the plants will be stronger in spring even though no obvious interim effect has been seen.

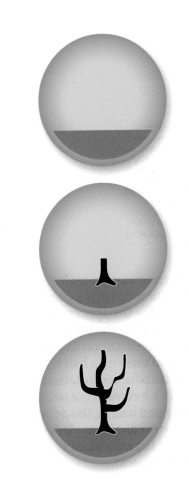

# The homeopathic consultation

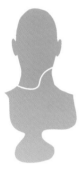

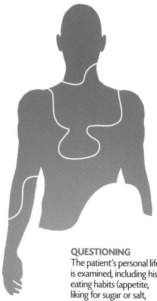

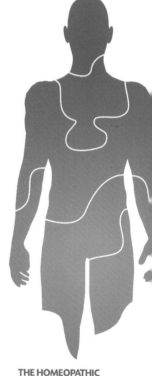

**LISTENING TO THE PATIENT**
This stage of the consultation covers all areas of the patient's past life, including background (medical and surgical history, accidents, psychological traumas), the family circle (relationships, recurring illnesses) and working conditions (rewarding, stressful).

**A** consultation with a homeopath is a gentle search for the appropriate medicine for the patient. The initial consultation can last around one and a half hours. A successful consultation is the link between the patient and good health, the point at which medical knowledge meets the individual's private world.

**QUESTIONING**
The patient's personal life is examined, including his eating habits (appetite, liking for sugar or salt, type of thirst and so on); reaction to climate (temperature, humidity, uncomfortable outdoors or indoors); stimulants (tobacco, alcohol, coffee, drugs); quality of sleep (sleeping position, getting up and going to sleep); body rhythm (periodic tiredness, need for a nap); behaviour (obsessive, fussy, disorganised); character (anxious, authoritarian, optimistic, calm, shy, enterprising); particular sensitivities (inability to tolerate smells or noises, lump in the throat, hollow feeling in the stomach); and emotions (nerves, temper, jealousy).

**THE HOMEOPATHIC DOCTOR'S EXAMINATION**
A medical doctor with homeopathic training may carry out a physical examination. This may include examination of nails and hair, weight and height, pulse, blood pressure, appearance, temperature of hands and feet, eyes (for irritation or sight problems) and oral health (appearance of the teeth and tongue).

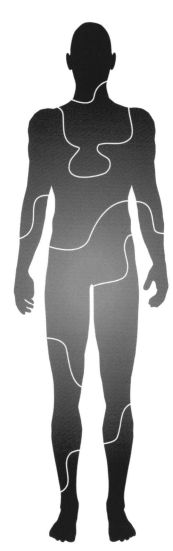

## FINDING THE RIGHT MEDICINE

Comparing all these elements to the *Medica Materia* will enable the homeopath to find the relevant medicine or medicines.

A homeopathic prescription can act on three levels: the constitution; the general condition at the time of the consultation; and the symptoms which were the reason for the visit. Thus the homeopath is not content simply to treat the latter, but also tries to tackle the cause of an imbalance or illness.

## WHAT ABOUT SELF-MEDICATION?

This is most suitable for acute illnesses; however regular appointments with a homeopath will help you to monitor your health and get to know yourself better. In the case of more established illnesses, it is advisable to consult your general practitioner or a qualified homeopath before taking any treatment. They will guide you and then gradually you will be able to treat certain everyday illnesses yourself.

### SUPPLEMENTARY TESTS

*The homeopathic doctor and qualified homeopath will normally carry out consultations slightly differently. The medically qualified doctor may carry out a clinical examination and recommend clinical tests (blood, urine, or investigative) as well as prescribing homeopathic medicines. The professional homeopath would listen carefully to the patient and prescribe a treatment, but suggest that the patient see a medical doctor if the condition appeared serious.*

# Allopathy and homeopathy

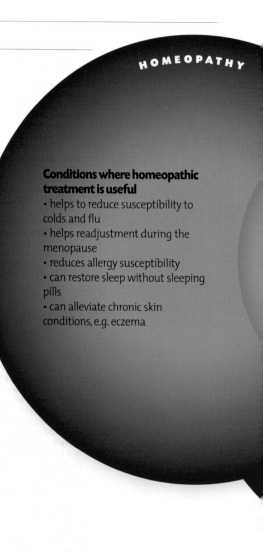

**H**omeopathy treats by mobilising the body's reactive capabilities and giving the body the ability to fight the illness itself. Allopathy was a term coined by Hahnemann to describe orthodox medicine. This type of medicine is described by homeopaths as providing the body with 'crutches' which act in its place when it is overloaded. Although homeopathy has no effect on irreversible conditions, homeopathy can increase the effectiveness of allopathic treatments and decrease their side effects.

**Conditions where homeopathic treatment is useful**
- helps to reduce susceptibility to colds and flu
- helps readjustment during the menopause
- reduces allergy susceptibility
- can restore sleep without sleeping pills
- can alleviate chronic skin conditions, e.g. eczema

## HAHNEMANN AND INOCULATIONS

*'Is it possible that cowpox inoculation protects against smallpox other than in a homeopathic manner?' asked Hahnemann. In fact, there are similarities between the vaccination process and the way homeopathy works, as both treat 'the disease with the disease'. Although initially in favour of vaccination, some homeopaths have since become reticent on this subject, as the doses used can sometimes create problems of their own such as side effects or even illness. In addition, vaccination fails to take account of the notion of constitution – everyone is treated in the same way.*

COMMON AREAS

**Conditions where a homeopath or GP may need to be consulted**
• treatment based on acute symptoms
• sore throats
• tonsillitis
• ear infections
• bronchitis
• sinusitis
• indigestion

**Allopathy or orthodox medicine**
Serious and life-threatening illnesses not treatable with homeopathy.
• illnesses caused by lesions (such as coronary thrombosis, acute appendicitis, fractures )
• serious hormonal problems (such as insulin-dependent diabetes, hyperthyroidism )
• illnesses requiring surgical intervention or serious medical intervention (such as chemotherapy radiotherapy, gene therapy)

PLEMENTARY TREATMENTS

**A complementary medicine**

When the patient's condition requires allopathic treatment, homeopathy can enable the doses to be reduced and lessen the side effects. The two can be combined in the treatment of many illnesses and also following surgery.

## HOMEOPATHY AND HERBALISM

As can happen with orthodox medicine the two therapies can be mutually exclusive (a herbalist's decoction of meadowsweet and willow bark would work against a homeopath's prescription of *Belladonna*). However, some combinations can prove beneficial. It is important to let practitioners know of other treatments you are receiving.

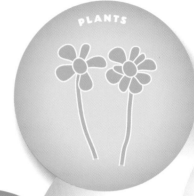

## HOMEOPATHY AND FOOD SUPPLEMENTS

It is entirely possible, even advisable, to combine homeopathy with trace elements, minerals and vitamins. In fact, the body reacts positively to treatments only if it is well maintained. If a vitamin, mineral or trace element is missing, it will respond badly. Well-targeted supplementation is thus useful. The trace elements are substances present in the body in very small but still measurable amounts which are essential to the enzymatic reactions of the cells.

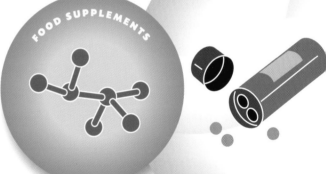

## HOMEOPATHY AND ALLOPATHY

There is no contraindication to prevent several therapies being combined, but they must be compatible. In the case of fever, there is no point in taking a homeopathic medicine to lower the temperature if an allopathic treatment is already being used to this end. On the other hand, two types of medicine can be combined when they complement one another. This would be the case, for instance, with high blood pressure or hormonal deficiencies.

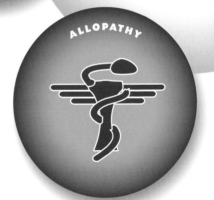

# Homeopathy – working with other therapies

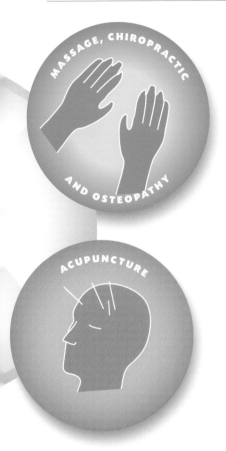

MASSAGE, CHIROPRACTIC AND OSTEOPATHY

ACUPUNCTURE

**H**omeopathy can be used alongside other therapies. Homeopaths always focus on the most beneficial combination of treatments for their patients. They may suggest osteopathy chiropractic, massage, acupuncture, herbal medicine, nutrition, to name a few, but will also recommend that patients see their general practitioner if the condition is serious.

### HOMEOPATHY AND MANIPULATIVE MEDICINES

Manipulative medicines, such as osteopathy and chiropractic, treat the patient by aligning the body posture, in particular, the spinal column and joints. These procedures do not conflict with homeopathy because they act in a totally different way.

### HOMEOPATHY AND ACUPUNCTURE

Some homeopaths are also acupuncturists, since the two methods are totally complementary. Acupuncture aims to readjust the vital force in the patient's body, and homeopaths have a similar notion of a balancing mechanism or force. The two procedures concur in that they give the body a message which helps it promote its own healing.

# Self-medication and treating a child

**H**ere are some simple, but essential, rules for self-medication:

## The six keys to homeopathic prescription at home

**1.** There must be at least three specific indications (symptoms suggesting a specific treatment), for a medicine to take it with certainty.

**2.** Do not take five or six medicines at once: one or two, suited to the case, will be sufficient.

**3.** Repeat the doses frequently, initially every 10 or 15 minutes, then every half hour, until symptoms improve.

**4.** Space them out when improvement is seen and only recommence if symptoms reappear.

**5.** Stop treatment when everything is back to normal.

**6.** If there is no improvement after two or three days' treatment, this does not mean that homeopathy is not 'working', simply that the treatment is not suitable and it would be best to consult a homeopath or homeopathic doctor, who will be able to find the right medicine.

**NB** Before attempting any self-medication, be sure to read 'Important notice for the reader' on page 128.

*His nose is streaming, he sneezes repeatedly. His upper lip is red and inflamed and his eyes are watering. Things seem better in the fresh air and worse in an overheated bedroom.*

**Give three pills of *Allium cepa* 6 c, as sneezing occurs.**

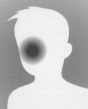

**MY CHILD HAS A RUNNY NOSE**

*The discharge has become greeny-yellow. Not really irritating, it is accompanied by shivers up and down the spine. The child alternates between anxious restlessness and exhaustion. His condition is worse at night in a warm bedroom.*

**1 pill of *Mercurius solubilis* 6 c, given 5 to 6 times a day, will improve his condition in a maximum of 3 days.**

It was a good party; the children played a lot and got very hot. When we got home, my little girl was subdued, her cheeks were red, wet with perspiration, she was exhausted. Her temperature was 39.5°C (103°F).

1 pill of *Belladonna* 6 c, every 15 minutes for 1 hour will allow the child to sleep and wake up fresh and full of energy the next day.

This morning everything was normal, but she got cold at playtime and came home from school shivering, excited and anxious. She slept after a light meal, but woke around 11 pm, agitated, pale and frightened, with a temperature of 40°C (104°F), but with no other symptoms.

1 pill of *Aconite* 6 c, repeated two or three times until asleep will control the problem during the night.

**MY CHILD HAS A TEMPERATURE**

This child is coming down with something! Sometimes pale, sometimes flushed, she seems slow, anxious, clammy: she has a slight temperature of 38.5°C (101°F).

1 pill of *Ferrum phosphoricum* 6 c, twice daily for 2 or 3 days, will put her back on her feet.

It's one o'clock in the morning! The child is crying, wakes up the whole house, anxious, upset then prostrate . He complains about his ear, which might have a discharge or bad smell. A bit of local warmth soothes him, he asks for cold water, then rejects it immediately.

1 pill of *Arsenicum album* 6 c, repeated often, will ease the pain.

**MY CHILD HAS EARACHE**

A violent pain, which appears in the throat, bronchial tubes, stomach or urinary tract, then settles in the ear, accompanied by a feeling of burning and tightness. The child wants to drink cold water, even though it makes him shiver. Warmth seems to soothe him.

1 pill of *Capsicum* 6 c continuously at first, then spaced out as the pain occurs, will quickly calm him.

# Treating an adult

**H**omeopathy is not just concerned with symptoms, but also the individual's reaction. It is these particular signs, developed by adults leading an active life, which enable the right medicine to be found and adapted to each life style.

(See also the six rules on page 84 and 'Important notice for the reader' on page 128.)

*Suddenly, your cheeks start to burn. You can feel the heat in the palms of your hands and the soles of your feet. A migraine attack begins with pain from the nape of the neck to just above the right eye. Fresh air doesn't help.*

*Sanguinaria 9 c, at each attack, will make the attacks less intense and decrease their frequency.*

*Since you turned 50, your body thermostat seems to have gone wrong. Your hands often feel red-hot and your feet are so hot at night that you have to put them outside the covers. You sometimes feel warmth on the crown of your head, or a general burning sensation. You perspire and the odour annoys you, because it seems to have changed.*

*1 pill of Sulphur 9 c at each attack will sort things out.*

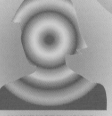

**I HAVE HOT FLUSHES**

*Suddenly feverish, your eyes and face are red. You are hot and can feel your head pounding. Your mouth is dry. Your whole body is hypersensitive. You feel better with rest and warmth.*

*1 pill repeated of Belladonna 6 c, repeated will improve the general condition.*

Between the worries, annoyances and heavy workload, you feel that you are falling apart. You go from long sighs to hysterical laughter and then to tears. You cannot tolerate strong smells, particularly other people's; a lump in the throat prevents you drinking, but disappears if you swallow a piece of bread.

1 pill of *Ignatia* 30 c, can give short term relief.

No sooner has the alarm gone off than you have to make breakfast, drop the children off at school, post that letter, think about this morning's meeting, fill your car with petrol. You hate being late and you start panicking which results in shaking and diarrhoea.

1 pill of *Argentum nitricum* 30 c will help but consult your homeopath for long term relief.

**I AM SUFFERING FROM STRESS**

You are inundated with work and yet you can't get going. The idea of getting started paralyses you. You then feel angry, which leaves you worn out and trembling. As for public speaking, the very idea of it is a nightmare!

1 pill of *Gelsemium* 30 c in the morning and when a mental block occurs will help you to feel more on top of things.

A yellowy complexion, a bad taste in the mouth and furred tongue, discomfort on the right-hand side, a hollow feeling in the stomach, constipation alternating with diarrhoea. Your stomach feels upset after a party. Only hot drinks (particularly lemon or milk) can soothe you.

*Chelidonium* 6 c, for 4 to 5 days, before each meal will relieve the symptoms.

**I'VE GOT INDIGESTION**

You enjoy life but you eat and drink too much. So you suffer from wind, flatulence and slow digestion. A little nap sorts things out, or even vomiting or passing a stool, but you suffer from constipation and wonder if you have haemorrhoids.

1 dose of *Nux vomica* 30 c can help ease your indigestion.

# Treating an elderly person

(See also the six rules on page 84 and 'Important notice for the reader' on page 128.)

The end of working life often leaves a lot of free time and minor irritations can take on greater significance. However, why let yourself be overwhelmed by run-of-the-mill problems which can ultimately spoil your life? Listen to your body and take action: this is a principle of homeopathy, which applies to all ages.

*In the morning, your joints feel as though they are rusty and are even worse when the weather is cold and rainy. Things improve during the day but as soon as you stop moving the pain returns and your spirits fall.*

**1 pill of *Rhus tox*. 6 c when you get up and during the day as the pain occurs, will ease your joints and lift your spirits.**

**I SUFFER FROM RHEUMATIC PAIN**

*In the warmth of your bed, everything is fine, but as soon as you get up, you feel as though you are carrying the worries of the world. Your hands, elbows, knees, back, sides and joints are red, swollen and hot. Firm pressure on the painful area brings relief, but the least movement causes a searing pain.*

**Bryonia 6 c repeated often will act like an anti-inflammatory drug, but without damaging your stomach.**

Although you don't really have anything to worry about, you can't stop thinking – about your children, your finances, your next holiday – and you can't sleep. The least sound disturbs you. You toss and turn which triggers an unbearable headache.

1 pill of *Coffea tosta* 6 c at bedtime, repeated when you wake during the night, will get rid of this type of insomnia.

Over anxious, you feel you are wasting away if you don't sleep. You are exhausted, agitated and frozen. Warmth helps you sleep but you wake at one o'clock in the morning and start to toss and turn and then you can't get back to sleep.

1 pill of *Arsenicum album* 6 c at bedtime and when anxious, taken regularly, will enable you to decrease and then stop taking your sleeping pills.

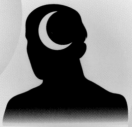

**I'M SLEEPING VERY BADLY**

With time, you are gradually losing your resilience. You ache, you are sensitive to everything around you, you worry about insecurity, violence, war and famine but feel powerless to act. You sometimes urinate whilst coughing or laughing.

1 pill of *Causticum* 6 c may help temporarily but consult your GP or a homeopath for further treatment.

**I'M DEPRESSED**

Everything feels heavy, you feel exhausted and wish your family would go away and leave you alone. You keep on weeping but don't know why and only lots of exercise makes you feel better.

*Sepia* 6 c morning and evening for a few days may help.

# Treating an animal

**W**hy should our favourite companions be left to suffer? Although they can't talk, their behaviour and attitude can speak for them instead. By learning to watch them, we can understand them better and treat them more effectively. But remember to consult your vet if a problem is serious or does not respond readily to the homeopathic medicine you have given. Alternatively, consult a homeopathic veterinary surgeon.

Suddenly shivery and sensitive to the cold, the cat curls up and rubs his eyes with his paw. Although his nose does not run, it might bleed, especially in a very warm room.

1 pill of *Dulcamara* 6 c, several times a day, will help him to recover.

A sudden high temperature leaves him exhausted from the heat and shaking. His head feels hot. He sneezes a lot and his nose streams causing irritation around his muzzle.

1 pill of *Gelsemium* 6 c should be given immediately and repeated at least 4 times daily.

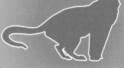

MY CAT HAS A HEAD COLD

Usually so calm and cuddly, my cat becomes irritable and cannot tolerate fresh air. He eats and drinks more than usual, but is constipated. He likes warm, secluded rooms, where he can be left in peace.

1 pill of *Bryonia* 6 c, several times daily will bring him back to normal, if the treatment is started early on in the illness.

(See also the six rules on page 84 and 'Important notice for the reader' on page 128.)

My dog can't stand any form of transport, he is even sick in a lift.

1 pill of *Borax* 9 c the day before departure, then 6 c every hour during the journey.

No matter what the method of transport we use, he feels ill. He lies still and silent, perhaps to prevent nausea. We can't open the window, because the fresh air seems to make him worse.

1 pill of *Cocculus indicus* 9 c the day before departure and 6c every hour during the journey.

**MY DOG IS SICK IN THE CAR/MY DOG CANNOT TOLERATE THE CAR**

As soon as he gets hot or moves, my dog is violently sick. His extremities are cold and strangely, he seems better when he closes his eyes. Driving with the window wide open soothes him.

1 pill of *Tabacaum* 9 c the day before departure and 6c every hour during the journey.

Inflammation of the tendon accompanied by muscular cramp. My horse is weak. He generally has brittle joints. Any sustained effort causes sprains and dislocations.

1 pill of *Natrum carbonicum* 9 c given every hour may result in him walking normally again.

**MY HORSE HAS TENDONITIS**

After a sudden strain, he suffers from inflammation of the tendon. His lameness disappears when he is moving and especially when it is rubbed, but his condition is worse in humid weather.

1 pill of *Rhus tox* 9 c every hour will bring effective relief.

My horse has tendonitis and looks sad and depressed. His tendon is retracted and feels deformed and he won't let us touch it. In fact, he seems worse if a hand is placed on the painful area. Only cold compresses soothe him

1 pill of *Gaïacum* 9 c every hour will quickly help him to get better.

# The ten basic homeopathic medicines

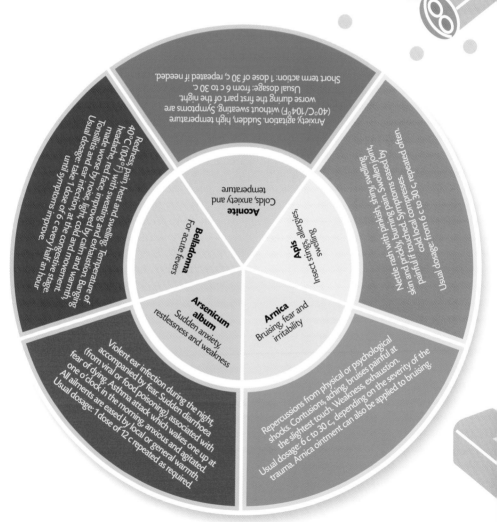

**Aconite**
Colds, anxiety and temperature

**Belladonna**
For acute fevers

**Apis**
Insect stings, allergies, swelling

**Arsenicum album**
Sudden anxiety, restlessness and weakness

**Arnica**
Bruising, fear and irritability

Anxiety, agitation. Sudden, high temperature (40°C/104°F) without sweating. Symptoms are worse during the first part of the night. Usual dosage: from 6 c to 30 c. Short term action: 1 dose of 30 c, repeated if needed.

Redness, pain, heat and swelling. 40°C (104°F) with sweating and headache, red face, improved by calm and exhaustion. Temperature of Tonsillitis and ear infection, light, cold and warmth. Banging headache. Temperature made worse by noise. Usual dosage: take 1 dose of 6 c at the congestive stage, until symptoms improve and movement, every half an hour.

Nettle rash with pinkish, shiny, swelling. Swollen joint, skin and prickly, burning pain. Symptoms eased by painful if touched cold local compresses. Usual dosage: from 6 c to 30 c, repeated often.

Repercussions from physical or psychological shocks. Contusions, aching bruises painful at the slightest touch. Weakness, exhaustion. Usual dosage: 6 c to 30 c, depending on the severity of the trauma. Arnica ointment can also be applied to bruising.

Violent ear infection during the night, accompanied by fear. Sudden diarrhoea (from viral or food poisoning), associated with fear of dying. Asthma attack which wakes one up at one o'clock in the morning, anxious and agitated. All ailments are eased by local or general warmth. Usual dosage: 1 dose of 12 c repeated as required.

**S**lowly but surely is the best approach when using homeopathic medicines for the first time. It is better to know how to use two or three medicines well than to get bogged down in dozens of remedies. Then, little by little, you can increase your range. Here are ten basic medicines, chosen to cover the most common ailments

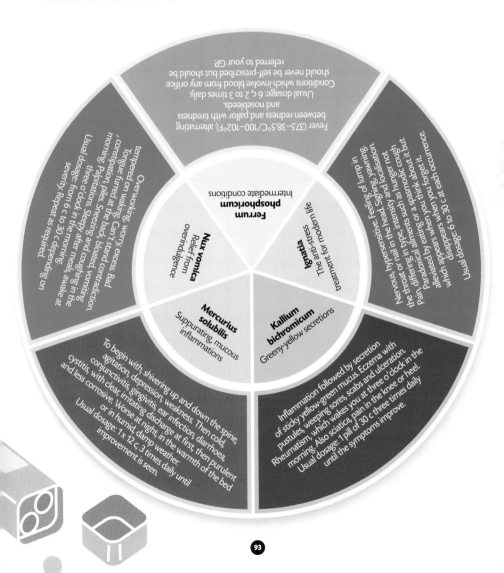

**Ferrum phosphoricum**
Intermediate conditions

Fever (37.5–38.5°C/100–102°F), alternating between redness and pallor with tiredness and nosebleeds.
Usual dosage: 6 c, 2 to 3 times daily.
Conditions which involve blood from any orifice should never be self-prescribed but should be referred to your GP.

**Nux vomica**
Relief from overindulgence

Overworking, worry, excess. Bad tempered on waking. Tongue furred at the back, constipation, piles. Sneezing and coughing in the morning. Palpitations, bloated, vomiting. Can't stand contradiction. Usual dosage: from 6 to 30 c depending on three o'clock in the morning, awake at severity. Repeat as required. Sleepy after meals,

**Ignatia**
The anti-stress treatment for modern life

Nervous, hypersensitive. Feeling of lump in the throat or nail in. Sighing, yawning, intensity and localisation. Pain differing in type, as hunger not a spasmodic cough but which appears when you forget it. Paradoxical ailments such as at each occurrence, alleviated by eating or you think about it. Usual dosage: 6 to 30 c disappears when you

**Mercurius solubilis**
Suppurating, mucous inflammations

To begin with, shivering up and down the spine, agitation, depression, weakness. Then cold, conjunctivitis, gingivitis, ear infection, diarrhoea, cystitis, with clear irritating discharge at first, then purulent and less corrosive. Worse at night, in the warmth of the bed or in humid, damp weather.
Usual dosage: 7 x 12 c, 3 times daily until improvement is seen.

**Kalium bichromicum**
Greeny-yellow secretions

Inflammation followed by secretion of sticky yellow-green mucus. Eczema with pustules, weeping sores, scabs and ulceration. Rheumatism, which wakes you at three o'clock in the morning. Also sciatica, pain in the knee or heel.
Usual dosage: 1 pill of 30 c three times daily until the symptoms improve.

# Types of homeopathic medicine

**H**omeopathic medicines can be produced in different forms, the most common in Britain being pills or granules.

### I. Pills

Pills can be hard or soft. Hard pills consist of 50 per cent sucrose (sugar) and 50 per cent lactose (milk-sugar), while soft pills are 100 per cent lactose. Drops of medicating potency are added to the bottles of pills to produce medicated pills which are then packed into small tubes.

### 2. Coarse granules

Smaller than the pills, these sucrose granules are more commonly used for the treatment of babies and children.

### 3. Gels and ointments

Specific dilutions can be mixed with the substances that are used for skin creams and gels. The main constituents can then penetrate through the skin.

### 4. Compounds

There is a growing number of homeopaths in the UK who prescribe compounds. This combination of substances is believed to produce a greater effect on a symptom and facilitates self-prescribing. For instance, the compound *Hamamelis*, used in venous circulatory disorders, is made from hamamelis, pulsatilla, echinacea and horse chestnut which all have an effect on this type of disorder.

### 5. Syrups

This type of medicinal product is particularly suited to winter ailments (cough, sore throat) and children. Homeopathic laboratories have devised syrups combining several dilutions.

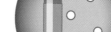

| HOW MUCH SUGAR? |
| --- |
| 1 sugar lump<br>= 5 grams of sucrose<br>= 55 pills<br>= 140 coarse granules |

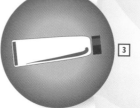

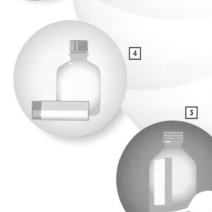

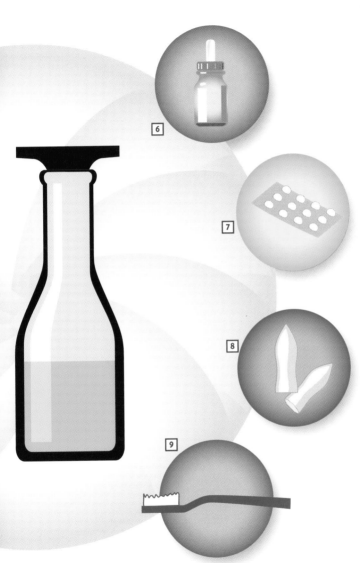

## 6. Drops

This traditional pharma-
ceutical form is still very
popular. Either the mother
tincture itself is used, or
a dilution or mixture of
several diluted substances.

## 7. Tablets

Tablets or pills are the
most common form of
homeopathic medicine in
Britain. Placed under the
tongue they are allowed to
dissolve for a few minutes
before being chewed and
swallowed.

## 8. Suppositories

Manufactured like
allopathic suppositories,
except that a homeopathic
dilution of one or more
substances is mixed with
the base product. Although
available in Britain from
specialist pharmacies, they
are rarely used.

## 9. Dental care

Nowadays there are
homeopathic toothpastes,
mouth rinses and even
chewing gum. The
dilutions they contain help
with the maintenance of
gum and tooth hygiene.

### DECIMAL DILUTIONS

*Certain compound
medicines contain decimal
dilutions (denoted by X
or D). They are obtained
in the same way as the
usual centesimals, except
for the addition of 1 drop
of product to 9 drops of
solvent at each stage.
Rarely used alone, they are
most often combined with
several other substances
and thus assist the action
of the higher dilutions.*

# Homeopathy across the globe

Homeopathy represents 0.4% of world pharmaceutical turnover, a figure of £650 million. A therapy of the future, homeopathy is proving increasingly popular throughout the world and its practice is growing more rapidly than that of conventional medicine.

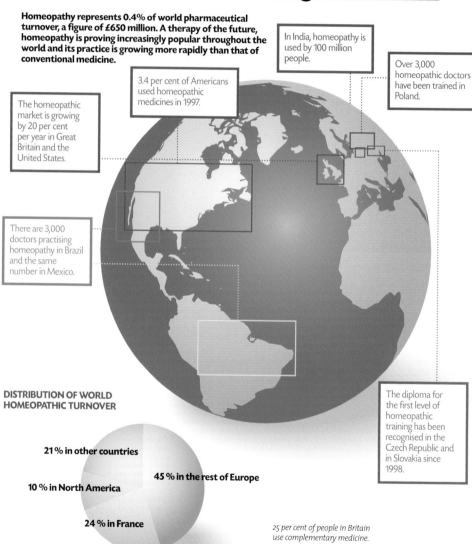

In India, homeopathy is used by 100 million people.

Over 3,000 homeopathic doctors have been trained in Poland.

3.4 per cent of Americans used homeopathic medicines in 1997.

The homeopathic market is growing by 20 per cent per year in Great Britain and the United States.

There are 3,000 doctors practising homeopathy in Brazil and the same number in Mexico.

The diploma for the first level of homeopathic training has been recognised in the Czech Republic and in Slovakia since 1998.

**DISTRIBUTION OF WORLD HOMEOPATHIC TURNOVER**

21 % in other countries

10 % in North America

45 % in the rest of Europe

24 % in France

*25 per cent of people in Britain use complementary medicine.*

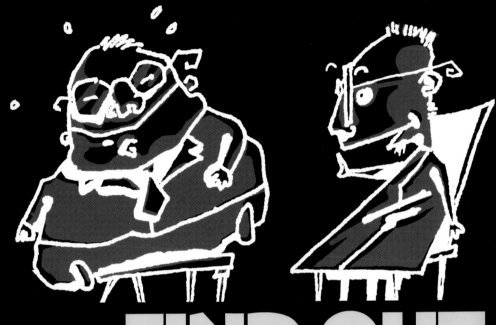

# FIND OUT

NO ONE HAS YET SUCCEEDED IN ESTABLISHING EXACTLY HOW HOMEOPATHY WORKS. EACH MEDICINE IS DESCRIBED AS HAVING A MATCHING PHYSICAL OR PSYCHOLOGICAL PORTRAIT. OFTEN, JUST TWO OR THREE HOMEOPATHIC MEDICINES IN THE FAMILY MEDICINE CHEST CAN HELP SOLVE A VARIETY OF PROBLEMS. ALL THAT REMAINS IS TO FIND A 'GOOD' HOMEOPATH OR HOMEOPATHIC DOCTOR, IN ORDER TO TREAT ILLNESSES THAT ARE MORE PROBLEMATIC.

# Water has a memory

**Homeopathy has been a subject of argument since its discovery. The debate is often conducted in scientific journals and occasionally even creeps into the national press. The controversy over the 'memory of water' is an example of a scientific quarrel which was widely publicised in 1988.**

## From dream to suspicion

On 30 June 1988 an article appeared in the British journal *Nature* under the obscure title 'Human basophil degranulation produced by very high dilutions of an anti-IGE antidote'. The studies were led by Dr Jacques Benveniste, the director of a unit at the French National Institute of Medical Research (INSERM) in Clamart, France, and a specialist in the immuno-pharmacology of allergies and inflammation. Three laboratories, in Revhot (Israel), Milan and Toronto, took part in the experiments and each came to the same extraordinary conclusion, a blood cell (basophil) can be activated by a simple aqueous solution containing an antibody diluted to the extreme. In other words, water can transmit a specific biological message and produce a molecular effect in the molecule's absence. Fifteen days before its publication in Nature, Jacques Benveniste had first described this phenomenon to a homeopathic congress in Strasbourg. 'It's as though water remembers having seen the molecule,' he said. The press crystallised the image: 'the memory of water'. Gone was the old notion of 'basophil degranulation'. The world's most common liquid, symbol of life, baptism and purity, was apparently endowed with a memory. Water never forgets. Yet if Dr Benveniste's statement was correct, it would mean that two centuries of learning in the field of physics and molecular biology would be overturned. It seemed that there might be a new higher level at which matter was organised.

The concept of the 'memory of water' was exciting for the lay person but it also threatened conventional science. Science is a field which has logically and consistently built up a proven body of knowledge, a series of great minds has, generation after generation, contributed to the development of molecular theory. The work of Benveniste threatened to turn this steady progress on its head. Could water retain the trace – and the active constituent – of something which no longer existed? When *Nature* decided to publish Jacques Benveniste's text (after two years' deliberation), the journal's chief editor at the time, John Maddox, added an editorial commentary entitled 'When to believe in the unbelievable.'

In his eyes, such a disruption in scientific theory requires 'more close questioning than usual as to whether or not the observation is correct'. With the passing of time, this little sentence began to sound like a preordained judgement. 'I was condemned by *Nature*,' said Jacques Benveniste, who has been ostracised by the scientific community ever since. In 1989, however, a renowned researcher came to Jacques Benveniste's rescue. Since *Nature* had refuted Dr Benveniste's analyses, Alfred Spira suggested that he would investigate

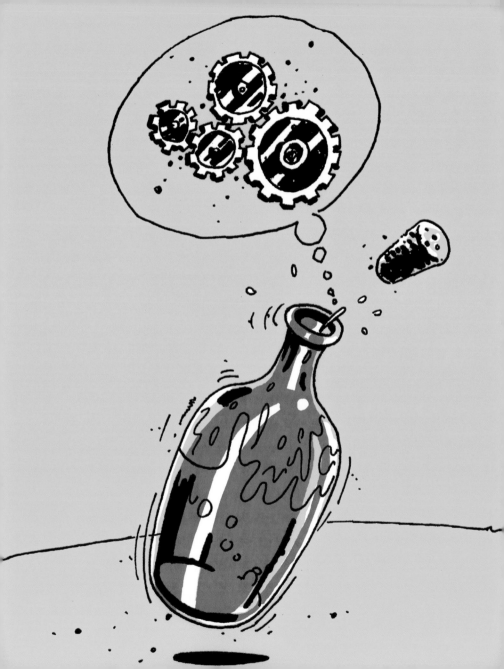

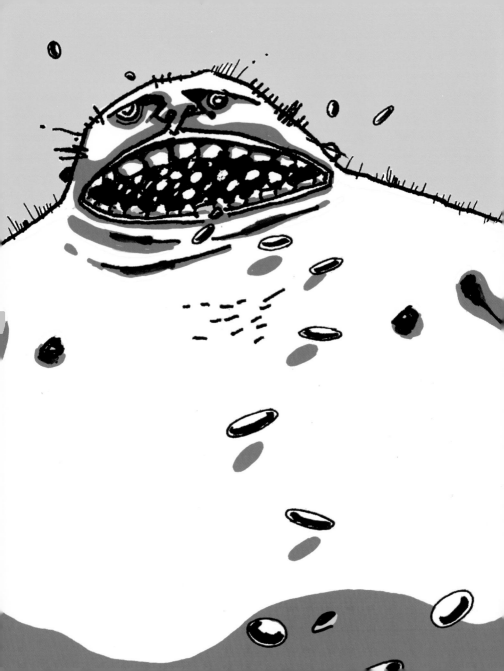

Benveniste's calculations. In an opinion column in the French newspaper, *Le Monde*, Spira justified his involvement. 'When a researcher asks questions which challenges established thinking, he is doing his job. To try and prevent him continuing his investigations when he has not been proved wrong is an indefensible restriction of his – and our – freedom. I shall thus continue to work with Benveniste, while we attempt to prove whether his results are false or accurate.'

## Passions aroused in the medical world

In an article in the French medical newspaper, *Quotidien du Medecin* of 4 April 1995, Dr Benveniste threatened: 'To deny my results is to insinuate fraud which, if made public, would lead to immediate libel proceedings.' In response to accusations by the Nobel prizewinning physicist, Georges Charpak, he gave this vexed and lofty reply, 'My feeling towards you borders on pity ... It is in fact a pity to see that you are unable to recognise how high the stake is.' He brought the issue to the attention of President Chirac of France in June 1996, arguing that it was more important than Lindbergh's cross-Atlantic flight. However, his opponents continued to put forward the same argument against him: 'Science is universal. The results achieved at Clamart must be repeatable elsewhere.'

## A highly diluted truth

Apart from the accusations of fraud, no other hypothesis on the structure of water arising from Benveniste's results has been put forward by competent researchers. When Benveniste presented his biological experiments to the French National Assembly, his speech was relayed over the Internet, but he was greeted with a polite silence from the scientific community, 'not one single question, not even a simple "what's it all about?".

Benveniste is perceived by his peers as a man who could cause scandal and provoke an outcry over the pseudo-sciences, beginning with homeopathy, but also bringing such diverse activities as hypnotism and witchcraft into the debate. Dr Benveniste is paying the price for all those charlatans who have tried to invade the scientific domain. By opting for the route of the mass media (though little other choice was open to him), he hastened his own downfall. Yet official science cannot accuse him of obscurantism, as he is not pursuing a particular personal interest but is attempting to make progress in the field of scientific investigation.

Benveniste does not claim to have brilliant intuition or a quick mind. 'I am a scientist, therefore I don't think,' he once said to underline that his observations are based, above all, on experiments which are 'honest and genuine yet produce inexplicable results'. They are not based on pre-existing ideas. Benveniste is not like the friar Gregor Mendel who, to support his 'premonition' about heredity, rigged his experimental results. Nor, however, is he a Galileo or a Pasteur, each of whom brought about a drastic reformulation of scientific truth – for no one can yet prove whether he is right or wrong. Nothing, within the current body of knowledge, predisposes scientists to accept Benveniste's proposal. Since 1988, things have moved on. The fraud accusations remain unsubstantiated and Benveniste continues his investigations into what he calls 'digital biology'. The possibility of artifice remains, but at the same time, the possibility also exists that Benveniste's work might have uncovered a new scientific truth.

© Eric Fottorino, *Le Monde*, 21, 22, 23 January 1997.)

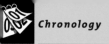

# Homeopathy's key dates

**1778** Hahnemann qualifies as a doctor.

**1790** Hahnemann discovers the 'law of similars' by taking cinchona bark.

**1796** Hahnemann's first essay and the official birth of homeopathy.

**1808** Hahnemann coins the term 'homeopathy'.

**1810** First publication of the Organon of the Healing Art.

*Constantin Hering*

**1813** Following Napoleon's campaign in Russia, Hahnemann treats the retreating French armies whose soldiers are suffering from typhus and cholera.

**1827** Frederick Hervey Quin and P. Curie introduce homeopathy to England.

**1830** Sébastien Des Guidi introduces homeopathy to France.

**1832** Quin sets up a London homeopathic practice. Korsakov creates his dilution method.

**1833** Hering introduces homeopathy to the United States.

**1835** Hahnemann marries a young French woman, Mélanie d'Hervilly and settles in Paris.

**1837** The first British homeopathic hospital is opened in Liverpool.

**1843** Hahnemann dies in Paris and is buried in the Père-Lachaise cemetery.

*Benoît Mure*

**1844** Quin establishes the British Homeopathic Society (later the Faculty of Homeopathy). The London Homeopathic Hospital is opened in Golden Square.

**1870**
Creation of the first homeopathic hospital in Paris, the Saint-Jacques hospital.

**1877**
Quin establishes the London School of Homeopathy (later the London Homeopathic Hospital and School of Medicine).

**1890**
The Tunbridge Wells Homeopathic Hospital is founded.

**1909**
The Homeopathic Association is founded in Britain to promote the knowledge and study of homeopathy.

**1914**
The Glasgow Homeopathic Hospital is founded.

**1920**
The London Homeopathic Hospital receives royal patronage.

**1925**
The Bristol Homeopathic Hospital is founded.

**1948**
The National Health Service is set up in Britain with provision for homeopathic treatment. An Act of Parliament establishes the Faculty of Homeopathy for doctors and other health care professionals. The Homeopathic Research and Educational Trust is founded to pursue education and research.

**1968**
The Hahnemann Society is founded in Britain to foster knowledge of homeopathy and support medical professionals who use homeopathy.

**1986**
First publication of homeopathic clinical research in the *Lancet*.

**1988**
Publication of the works of Jacques Benveniste in *Nature*, at the start of the 'memory of water' debate.

**1992**
Publication of a European directive on homeopathic medicines.

**1997**
The European Commission orders a study into homeopathy.

Samuel Hahnemann

Sébastien Des Guidi

# Which homeopathic remedy profile fits you?

**During his experiments, Hahnemann carefully noted the physical and psychological reactions produced by substances on healthy subjects and constructed, for each homeopathic medicine, a remedy picture. We rarely correspond totally to a single medicine, yet we can perhaps recognise some of the traits, which may indicate that the medicine will suit us. Study these twelve profiles carefully: perhaps you will recognise yourself, or someone you know.**

### Argentum nitricum: the person in a hurry

She never has enough time, there are too many things to do, making her irritable, anxious, even distressed. This makes her almost phobic, afraid of crowds, loneliness, open spaces and particularly heights, because she is attracted by the fall. Prone to stage fright, which makes her even more anxious. Public speaking terrifies her and she may suffer diarrhoea, indigestion and belching.
•A dose of Argentum nitricum 12 c will restore her confidence.

### Arsenicum album: the anxious perfectionist

Even when he's well, he's worried: something must be wrong. He is afraid of death, believes he is suffering from an incurable disease and thus devises plans to cover all eventualities. He is always punctual and careful with money. His 'sickness' is behavioural, he checks that he's turned the cooker off ten times before going out and that his keys really are in his pocket, obsessive actions which temporarily reassure him. He is very sensitive to the cold and avoids draughts. He is prone to chronic, recurring infections such as asthma, allergies or eczema.

Things seem worse between 1 and 3 am in the morning.
• A dose of Arsenicum album 6 c will enable him to get back to sleep.

### Gelsemium sempervirens: paralysed by stage fright

Fears include having only a blank sheet of paper and unexpected memory failure. She is totally incapable of getting on with things, which annoys her. She becomes inhibited and feels trapped in a stupor. If forced into action, she begins to tremble, unable to utter a word and runs for the toilet, afflicted by diarrhoea which leaves her prostrate.
• Gelsemium 12 c gets rid of inhibitions and can be taken as often as required.

### Ignatia amara: stressed

Home, work, family and friends can all cause stress and overwork. He acts with great haste, and is anxious, to the point where his reactions are uncontrollable and he becomes hypersensitive. He is a paradoxical creature, like a smoker who can't stand the smell of other people's tobacco. This produces spasms:

the feeling of a lump in his throat or an empty stomach, uncontrollable yawning and an acute headache. Things improve if he can be entertained.
• Ignatia amara 12 c can provide short term relief. Discuss a long-term cure with your homeopath.

## Lachesis muta: the chatterbox

This well-dressed woman of around fifty will bury you in her avalanche of words which can go on and on. She is frequently too hot and needs space and air. She is uncomfortable in a lift or airplane. A necklace can make her more uncomfortable and increase her hot flushes. The slightest impact bruises her (great capillary weakness).
• Lachesis 6 c or 12 c, 3 during a crisis or hot flush will improve all the symptoms.

## Lycopodium clavatum: the family tyrant

This model, intelligent pupil annoys his teachers with incessant, but relevant questions. At home, he is bossy if allowed. As an adult, he is intransigent and despotic. In fact, he suffers from a terrible lack of self-confidence. He loves sugar, but this light eater does not like big meals. He suffers flatulence (he has to loosen his belt) and has slow digestion (at 6 o'clock, his lunch is still working its way through the body). As he gets older, his memory fails him and he becomes irritable, confused, gloomy, and even cantankerous.
• Lycopodium 6 c, repeated as needed for digestive problems.

## Natrum muriaticum: the thin depressive

Any psychological shock makes her lose weight. Stress also depletes her appetite and life forces. However, she likes to eat well, particularly very salty food. She catches everything including herpes, head colds and conjunctivitis and feels ill at ease. She may have 'wrinkly' or oily skin and suffers from eczema or acne. Everything weighs heavily on her, she has a feeling of pelvic weakness, incontinence and lumbago. Although sensitive to the cold, she nonetheless feels better in the fresh air but dreads the time of day when her energy levels drop, usually 10 o'clock in the morning.
• A dose of Natrum muriaticum 6 c, taken regularly, will help.

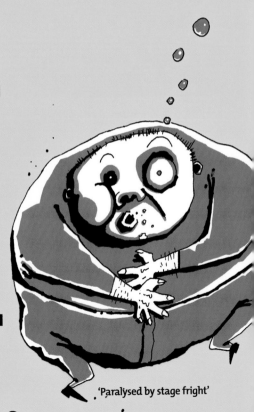

'Paralysed by stage fright'

## Nux vomica: the hyperactive boss

As a child, he won't stand still – running, playing, jumping, dragging along his friends, brothers and sisters. As an adult, he thrives on stimulation and is ambitious at home as well as at work. He likes stimulants: coffee, tobacco, alcohol. Good meals make him gain weight but he has neither the time nor the inclination to do any physical exercise. He can't tolerate contradiction provoking violent fits of anger, which quickly pass. A quick nap revives him and puts him back on his feet. As he gets older and more settled, he begins to find it difficult to get going in the morning, particularly following periods of insomnia at around 3 o'clock in the morning. He tends to go back to sleep when the alarm goes off, which puts him in a bad mood for the whole day. Nux vomica 6 c, when troubled, will help restore calm until the next time.

## Phosphorus: the lively, pleasant person

Elegant and stimulating, she loves being surrounded by people, talking, telling stories. However, she tires easily and soon feels as if her stomach is empty. She flares up and calms down quickly. She soon recovers after a good night's sleep. When she is ill, she feels a burning sensation in the throat, back or hands. Sensitive to the surrounding environment, she doesn't like storms and is depressed at twilight.
• Phosphorus 12 c, taken regularly, will help control her impressionable nature.

## Pulsatilla: the shy, hypersensitive person

As soon as a voice is raised, this shy child huddles up and clings to his mother's arm, his eyes filled with tears. Later in life, he finds it difficult to leave the family fold through fear of the unknown. Emotion makes him sweat (particularly his extremities, which are cold). Sometimes he finds it difficult to hold his pen during an exam or to shake hands with a stranger. The fresh air does him good. His mucous membranes are delicate, he suffers colds, bodily discharges and diarrhoea caused by greasy food. He shifts seamlessly from one state to another, from laughter to tears. His pleasant, fragile and resigned appearance may hide the kind of courage which demonstrates a will of iron.
• Pulsatilla 12 c can help get him back on his feet.

## Staphysagria: the frustrated obsessive

This sensitive type suppresses emotions. Her gestures can indicate that if you offend her she may become angry or melancholic. Sexually obsessive, her urogenital system is troublesome, often causing pain in the urinary tract without bacterial infection, although cystitis can be a problem. She can't tolerate injustice, and feels ill at ease, which causes an itching sensation in different parts of her body with verrucas, styes or weeping eczema.
• Staphysagria 12 c, repeated according to need will make life easier.

## Silicea: the irritable, undernourished person

Hypersensitive and irritable, he suffers from chronic suppurations of the nose, throat, ears, lungs, skin and bones and his digestion is poor. Shy, anxious, fainthearted, he has difficulty concentrating and is afraid of not being up to the task. He enjoys intellectual success, but this also exhausts him. Despite being sensitive to the cold, his head and particularly his feet are sweaty and he only feels well when warmly covered.
• Silicea 12 c will help him absorb nutrition.

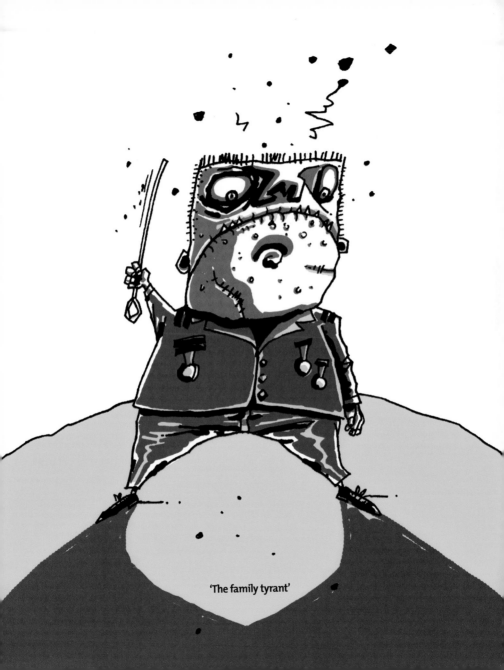

'The family tyrant'

# The homeopathic family medicine chest

**A few tubes of granules and ointment of the most common remedies, as advised by your homeopath, make up the ideal medicine chest.**

## Where to find homeopathic medicines

Homeopathic medicines are manufactured by specialist suppliers and homeopathic laboratories. They can be dispensed by professional homeopaths, or bought from health food shops and most high street chemists, as well as by mail order and through the Internet. Prescriptions supplied by NHS homeopathic hospitals are free while some private insurance schemes will refund the costs of homeopathic consultations and medicines. The specialist suppliers listed in this book (pp. 118–121) may be able to offer advice on specific remedies.

## Seeking advice from the chemist

Although every high street chemist is allowed by law to sell homeopathic medicines, not all of them will be able to offer advice. Here are a couple of precautions of which to be aware.
Don't confuse the potencies (ie do not replace the prescribed potency with another one: 6 c and 30 c are two different things).
Don't get the products mixed up – some have similar names such as China and Cina, Kalium bromatum and Kalium bichromicum.

## The homeopathic family medicine chest

This need contain only a few medicines as just a dozen or so homeopathic treatments can be used to treat many illnesses.
In particular, it should include those that you know how to use properly. The collection can also be expanded, with the help of your homeopathic practitioner, to include medicines suited to you that you will use regularly.

## Maintenance and storage

Homeopathic medicines should be stored in a dark, dry place away from strongly smelling substances such as aromatherapy oils, perfumes and toothpaste.

## Essential homeopathic products

Start with a basic first aid kit and add those medicines as recommended by your practitioner, that are specific to you and your family. Buy the following pills in 6 c, 12 c and 30 c to get started: Aconite, Apis, Arnica, Arsenicum album, Belladonna, Ignatia, Kali brichromicum, Mercurius solubilis, Nux vomica.

## Mother tinctures

These are available from specialist suppliers but they are not generally recommended for home use.

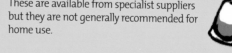

• Calendula mother tincture: antiseptic and healing, use a few drops in a little water to bathe a wound, or as an oral disinfectant.
• Phytolacca mother tincture: use a few drops in a glass of warm water, as a gargle, for a sore throat radiating towards the ears (can be combined with calendula).
• Echinacea mother tincture: a few drops on toothpaste can sooth inflamed gums.

## Gels and creams

These are useful and practical for treating minor cuts and bruises.
• Arnica gel: for bruises, shock, muscular pain.
• Apis gel: for insect bites.
• Calendula cream: for skin irritations.

**NB** See also the six rules on page 84 and 'Important notice for the reader' on page 128.

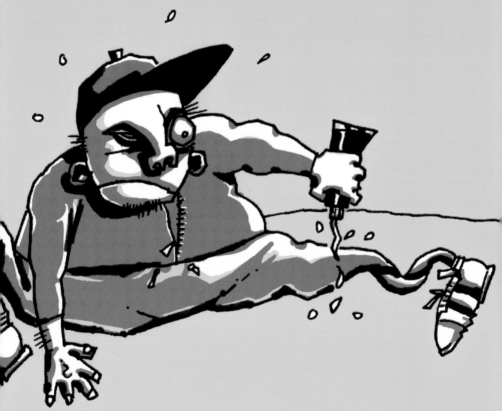

'Gels and creams are useful and practical for treating cuts and bruises.'

# Ten common ailments and their treatments

**Here are a few common and easily recognisable bodily symptoms. Nevertheless, don't forget to tell your homeopath about them.**

### 1. 'I've got a headache'

• Brought on by severe stress, the pain is piercing. You feel better when you are being entertained as it takes your mind off the problem. Ignatia 12 c, repeated until things improve.

### 2. 'I've got a cough'

• Tickling feeling in the larynx. Coughing fits which resemble whooping cough, but with thick, free-flowing mucus, which sometimes almost makes you vomit. Coccus cacti 6 c, following each attack.

### 3. 'My children feel sick'

• The tongue is pink, normal: Ipecac 6 c.
• The tongue is coated with white curd-like substance: Antimonium crudum 6 c.
• The tongue is pink on the tip and white at the back: Nux vomica 6 c.
Give a dose of the medicine shown and repeat as the nausea symptoms occur.

### 4. 'I'm constipated'

• It lasts several days. Feelings of distension and wind. Occasional bulky and painful stools which make you hold back. Graphites 6c, before every meal until digestion returns to normal.

• Frequent urge to defecate, but completely unproductive. Slow digestion. You enjoy life but get frequent upset stomachs and your tongue is furred at the back. Nux Vomica 6 c, as digestive symptoms appear.

### 5. 'I've got spots'

• Caused by an insect bite with a tendency to bleed and become infected. Ledum palustre 6 c, daily until healed.
• Urtica urens, after sunstroke, contact with an allergenic product or a wasp sting. Itching sensation improved by a local cold compress. Apis 6 c, every 10 minutes until the symptoms are eased.

### 6. 'I feel dizzy '

• Occurs when you turn your head, get back into bed or move your eyes. You feel physical and psychological weakness. You can't stand the light. Conium muculatum 6 c, repeated as necessary.

### 7. 'I've got a stiff neck'

• Pain predominantly on the right-hand side although it radiates to the nape and the head. Lachnantes tinctoria 6 c, 5 to 6 times daily and Arnica montana 6 c, 5 to 6 times daily (alternating).

• You have pain on swallowing and on touching the throat, which is red and feels like an open wound. However, eating brings relief. Arum triphyllum 6 c, as required until healed.

• Your whole body is cold, even your nose. Paradoxically, you can't stand being covered, you are exhausted, shivery, prostrate. Camphora 6 c, 3 or 4 times in succession. If taken when symptoms first appear, it may prevent the conventional cold which can last 15 days.

• Unbearable pain, causing agitation, irritability and a numb feeling. It is worse when you drink something hot. Chamomilla 6 c, repeated as necessary will be more effective than any chemical pain killer, without the side effects.

## Help your body

Homeopathy heals by remobilising your body, it reactivates your 'sleeping' healing forces. However it can only do this if your body is able to react. For this reason it would not be prescribed, for example, in the case of insulin-dependent diabetes or when major surgery is needed. However, it can help to speed recovery following surgery. To further improve the efficiency of homeopathic treatment, adopt a healthier life style: healthy eating and regular physical exercise.

## Help your homeopath

A successful homeopathic consultation relies on effective communication between the practitioner and yourself. It is recommended that you answer all the homeopath's questions, even if they seem strange. Learn to observe yourself, to see your reactions differently and examine your symptoms.

## Become more familiar with the ailment

**1. The time**
When does the disorder occur? Is it mainly in the morning or evening, during the day or night, at a particular time or during a particular season?

**2. The weather**
Is the ailment affected by the cold, heat, humidity, dry conditions, wind?

**3. The place**
Is it worse indoors or outdoors, by an open or closed window?

**4. The modalities (things that make the condition better or worse)**
Examine the condition in order to describe it in detail. Is the pain burning, prickly, dull, piercing, on the left or right hand side? Is the discharge, thin, thick, smelly, sticky?

**5. Any other details**
Note any details which occur to you, especially those which seem strange. They might help the homeopath to choose between several medicines, in order to find the one which most closely matches the symptoms described.

# How to find a good homeopath

**Finding a homeopath is one thing.
Finding one who really suits you is another.**

## Homeopathic training

Recognised training standards in Britain are set by the professional bodies. Training exists for medical professionals and, separately, for lay practitioners through a variety of private colleges. The Faculty of Homeopathy is the association for doctors and other healthcare professionals. It has five accredited training centres. Most of the private colleges are linked to the Society of Homeopaths, the association for professional homeopaths. The society has 2,500 members and is a member of the European and International Councils for Classical Homeopathy (ECCH and ICCH). Course length varies from a few weeks for medical professionals to three years full time or four years part-time. The University of Westminster is the only university to offer a degree course in homeopathy as part of a joint venture with the London College of Classical Homeopathy.

## What makes a good homeopath or homeopathic doctor?

A good homeopath or homeopathic doctor will have completed a recognised training course, is capable of listening to you and will take into account your current health problems and all the relevant details of your lifestyle and environment.

## How to choose a good homeopath?

The best homeopath is the one who suits *you*, and in whom you have confidence. He or she is, after all, someone you can contact in the case of an acute problem and whose treatment actually 'works'. If you don't feel totally happy in their presence, don't hesitate to find another practitioner.

The following are signs of a good practitioner:
• The amount of time it takes to see you: a short consultation should arouse suspicion. The first homeopathic consultation should last one and a half hours, perhaps more.
• Questioning: a homeopath asks questions which might seem remote from your problem, but which help to work out your temperament, susceptibility and reactions. Don't be surprised if the first consultation is quite different from that of any conventional doctor.
• The prescription: the homeopath aims to find the 'similarity' between you, your illness and the appropriate medicine. Although a prescription may not be restricted to a single medicine, it should, nonetheless, be short: more than four or five medicines for the same illness indicate that the homeopath does not have a very good 'grasp' of your problem.
• The explanation: a homeopath should be able to explain your prescription to you in detail.

## Plural, single or combination?

Most English homeopaths are classically trained, which means they look for the 'similar', the single remedy that can address all of the physical, emotional and mental symptoms by re-establishing the patient's internal balance. In France, most homeopaths are pluralists, often prescribing several medicines together. Homeopaths using combination remedies prescribe a formula combining different medicines, in low dilutions, to treat a specific ailment.

## Where to find a homeopath or homeopathic doctor

• By recommendation: ask your friends and family.
• By referral through your GP or through a professional association or users' group (see pp.118–119).

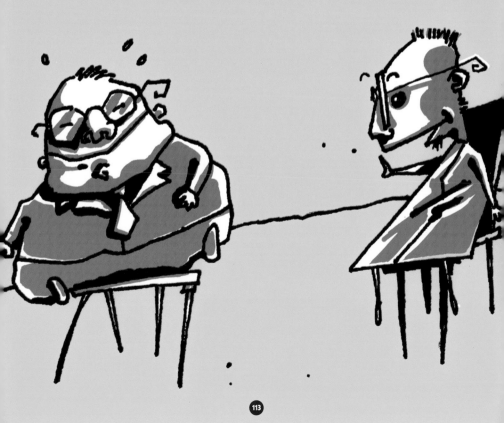

# Generally accepted ideas: true or false?

**1. You shouldn't take mint when you are using homeopathic treatment.**
**False**
A recent French study focused on the investigation of the possible effect of mint cordial on the anti-inflammatory action of *Apis 7 c* following the exposure of human guinea pigs to ultraviolet rays. The study concluded that the action of a homeopathic medicine is not affected by taking mint.

**2. You mustn't touch homeopathic medicines with your fingers.**
**False**
It was previously thought that the active product, impregnated from the outside, was left on the surface of the medicines and could thus remain on the fingers. French research has shown that the medicines are soaked through to the centre so touching them presents no risk.

**3. You shouldn't swallow the pills, but suck them slowly.**
**True**
Homeopathic medicines are rapidly absorbed through the numerous blood vessels which line the tongue and mouth.

**4. Homeopathy is a slow-acting medicine.**
**False**
Homeopathy's speed of action depends on the health problem in question. To treat an ear infection or a high temperature, just a few hours are required. To cure tonsillitis or flu takes several days. As a general rule, the more acute and recent an illness, the quicker it is cured by homeopathy. This is why it is important to act as soon as the symptoms appear, although in the case of chronic illnesses, treatment may take some time.

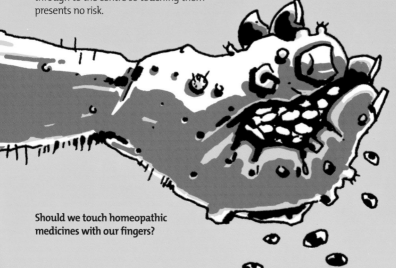

Should we touch homeopathic medicines with our fingers?

Nevertheless, any homeopathic treatment which has no effect after three or four weeks should be reconsidered, as this implies that the chosen medicines are unsuitable.

## 5. You have to believe in homeopathy for it to work.
**False**

For 20 years, veterinary medicine has contributed to the development of homeopathy because it has shown that the therapy works on animals which are unaware of what they are taking and therefore cannot be said to be subject to the placebo effect.

## 6. Homeopathy is a placebo.
**False**

Clinical studies have shown that homeopathy is statistically more effective than a placebo. It was homeopaths themselves who, from the beginning of the 20th century, developed the placebo principle to prevent the patient's beliefs from confusing the real effects of homeopathic medicine.

## 7. Homeopathy is completely safe.
**True and false**

Thanks to the small amount of product contained, homeopathy does not cause side effects. It can therefore be very useful during pregnancy, for babies and the elderly. However, homeopathic remedies are still active medicines. Do not take them indiscriminately as this could have undesired effects. For instance, in the case of a bodily discharge, the wrong dilution can make things worse, since a low dilution increases the discharge while a high dilution stops it.

## 8. Homeopathy is a medical speciality.
**True and false**

Homeopathy is a recognised medical specialty within the National Health Service but there is no statutory regulation of homeopaths in Britain as a whole. In practice, however, it is a real medical speciality, in that it requires a particular, global concept of the individual, separate from conventional medicine's perspective of the patient as a collection of 'parts'.

## 9. Homeopathy doesn't work for everyone.
**False**

In the case of an acute illness, if the treatment hasn't worked after 24 hours, change it. Either the dosage is too low or the medicine is wrong. Constitutional treatments take longer. If the treatments don't work, don't think it's because homeopathy is ineffective or doesn't work on certain people. Consult a homeopath who will be able to correct the prescription.

## 10. You must never give a homeopathic prescription to someone else.
**True**

Homeopathy is an individualised medicine. The choice of remedy depends on the patient and their reactions. This differs from one person to another for the same illness. A homeopathic remedy which does not take this into account cannot work. However, home prescription for simple complaints is an excellent way of making your friends and family aware of the efficacy of homeopathy.

# Homeopathy statistics

**The British are becoming more and more interested in this type of treatment. Homeopathic medicines cost little, compared to conventional drugs, although private consultations can be costly. The following figures show how the image of homeopathy is gradually changing.**

## Pharmaceutical industry

- Americans spent US$230 million on homeopathic medicines in 1996.
- It takes 12 days to make a globule, 16 days for a granule, 21 days for a mother tincture.
- Only 0.08 per cent of the NHS research budget is spent on complementary medicine.
- Sales of Nelson's homeopathic remedies grew to £25 million in 2000.
- Over-the-counter sales of homeopathic medicines are growing by 20 per cent every year.

## The social cost

- A survey of outpatients from the Royal London Homeopathic Hospital revealed that 29 per cent of patients had stopped taking their conventional medication and 33 per cent had decreased their usage.
- The average cost of a homeopathic prescription to the NHS is less than £2.

## Doctors

- In 1992 the journal for GPs, *Doctor*, conducted a survey of readers and found that 80 per cent of the GPs who responded, believed homeopathy to be effective.
- A Scottish study of the views of GPs on complementary therapies revealed that 69 per cent of those who responded had referred patients for homeopathy. The same study revealed that 37 per cent of GPs had some training in complementary therapies and 46 per cent wanted training, particularly in homeopathy.
- The Faculty of Homeopathy has a membership of around 1,000 doctors who may use the title MFHom.
- Between 1981 and 1998, the number of homeopaths registered with the Society of Homeopaths increased from 41 to 591. There are around 1,000 registered professional homeopaths in the UK today.
- In 1997 GP referrals to the Royal London Homeopathic Hospital increased by 31 per cent.
- A study published in the *British Medical Journal (BMJ)* noted that out of 100 recently graduated British doctors, 80 per cent expressed an interest in being trained in homeopathy and other complementary therapies.

## The patients

- 25 per cent of people in Britain use complementary medicine.
- A survey of a British consumer organisation showed that 80 per cent of its 28,000 members had used complementary medicine and 70 per cent said they were cured or improved by it.
- Studies of users of complementary medicine in Britain have shown that use is higher in women, the middle-aged, in the south and in higher socio-economic groups.

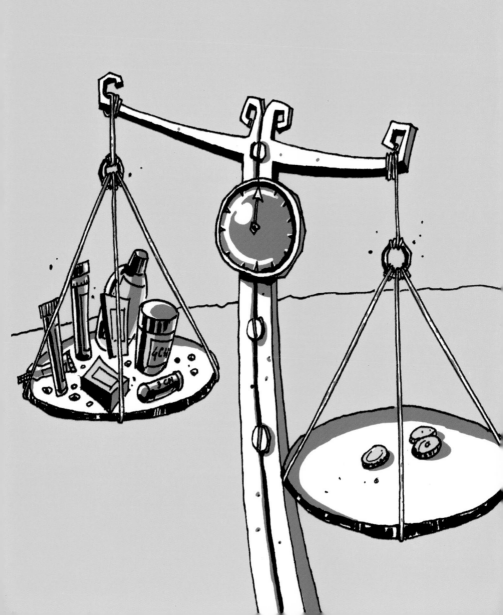

# Information and training

▼

## HOMEOPATHIC PRACTITIONER ORGANISATIONS

**BRITISH ASSOCIATION OF HOMEOPATHIC VETERINARY SURGEONS**
Alternative Veterinary Medicine Centre
Chinham House
Stanford-in-the-Vale
Faringdon
Oxon SN7 8NQ
Tel: 01367 710324
Website: www.bahvs.com

**BRITISH HOMEOPATHIC ASSOCIATION**
15 Clerkenwell Close
London ECIR OAA

**BRITISH HOMEOPATHIC DENTAL ASSOCIATION**
2b Franklin Road
Watford
Herts WD11QD
Tel: 01923 233 336
Tel: 020 7566 7800
Website: www.trusthomeopathy.org

**FACULTY OF HOMEOPATHY**
15 Clerkenwell Close
London EC1R OAA
Tel: 020 7566 7810
Website: www.homeopathy.org.uk

**THE HOMEOPATHIC MEDICAL ASSOCIATION**
6 Livingstone Road
Gravesend
Kent DA12 5DZ
Tel: 01474 560336
Website: www.the-hma.org

**INTERNATIONAL REGISTER OF CONSULTANT HERBALISTS AND HOMEOPATHS**
32 King Edward Rd
Swansea SA14LL
Tel: 01792 655886

**THE INTERNATIONAL REGISTER OF HOMEOPATHIC PRACTITIONERS**
32 King Edward Road
Swansea SA14LL
Tel: 01792 655886

**THE SOCIETY OF HOMEOPATHS**
2 Artizan Road
Northampton NNI 4HU
Tel: 01604 21400
Website: www.homoeopathy.org.uk

## NHS HOMEOPATHIC HOSPITALS

**BRISTOL HOMEOPATHIC HOSPITAL**
Cotham Hill
Cotham
Bristol BS6 6JU
Tel: 0117 731231

**DEPARTMENT OF HOMEOPATHIC MEDICINE**
Mossley Hill Hospital
Park Avenue
Liverpool L18 8BU
Tel: 0151 724 2335

**GLASGOW HOMEOPATHIC HOSPITAL**
1053 Great Western Road
Glasgow G12 OXQ
Tel: 0141 211 1600

**ROYAL LONDON HOMEOPATHIC HOSPITAL**
Great Ormond Street
London WC1N 3HR
Tel: 020 7837 8833

**TUNBRIDGE WELLS HOMEOPATHIC HOSPITAL**
Church Road
Tunbridge Wells
Kent TN11JU
Tel: 01892 542 977

## USERS AND PATIENTS ORGANISATIONS

**BRITISH HOMEOPATHIC ASSOCIATION**
27A Devonshire Street
London W1N 1RJ
Tel: 020 7935 2163
Website: www.trusthomeopathy.org

**THE BRITISH HAHNEMANN SOCIETY**
2 Powis Place
London WC1N 3HZ
Tel: 020 7837 3297

**INSTITUTE FOR COMPLEMENTARY MEDICINE**
PO Box 194
London SE16 7QZ
Tel: 020 7237 5165
Website: www.icmedicine.co.uk
*A registered charity formed to provide information on complementary medicine.*

## RESEARCH AND STUDY ORGANISATIONS

**THE HOMEOPATHIC RESEARCH AND EDUCATIONAL TRUST**
15 Clerkenwell Close
London EC1R OAA
Tel: 020 77566 7800

**THE RESEARCH COUNCIL FOR COMPLEMENTARY MEDICINE**
505 Riverbank House
1 Putney Bridge Approach
London SW6 3JD.
Tel: 020 7231 5770
Website: www.rccm.org.uk

## TRAINING

*Consult the Society of Homeopaths or the Homeopathic Medical Association for a full listing.*

**BRITISH INSTITUTE OF HOMOEOPATHY LIMITED**
Cygnet House
Market Square
Staines
Middx TW18 4RH
Tel: 01784 440467/466251

**THE COLLEGE OF PRACTICAL HOMEOPATHY**
760 High Road
North Finchley
London N12 9QH
Tel: 020 8445 6123

**THE COLLEGE OF HOMEOPATHY**
Regent's College Inner Circle
Regent's Park
London NW14NS
Tel: 020 7487 7416

**LONDON COLLEGE OF CLASSICAL HOMEOPATHY**
Hahnemann House
32 Welbeck Street
London W1M 7PG
Tel: 020 7487 4322
also
21 Abercombe Place
Edinburgh EH3 6QE
and
Aizlewood Business Centre
Aizlewood
Mill Nursery Street
Sheffield S3 8GG

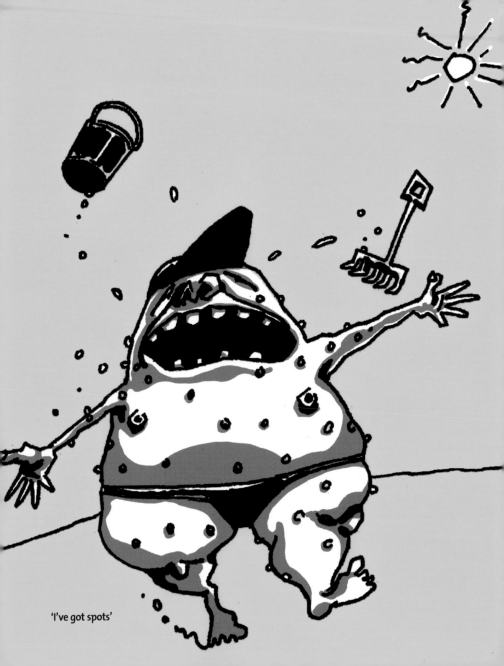

'I've got spots'

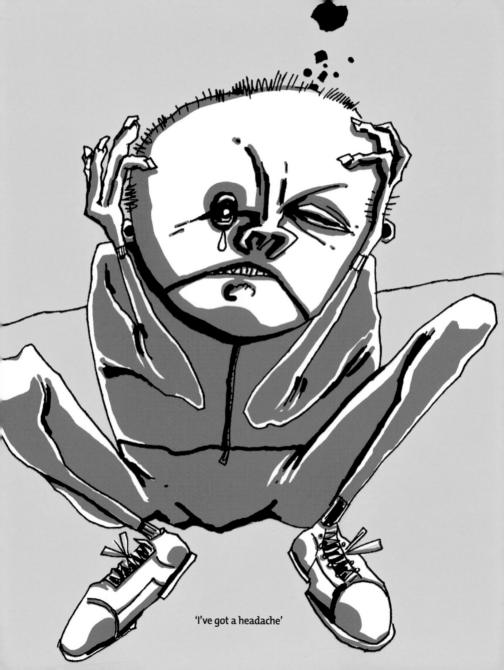

'I've got a headache'

**HAHNEMANN COLLEGE OF HOMEOPATHY**
164 Ballards Road
Dagenham
Essex RM10 9AB
Tel: 020 8984 9240

**THE LONDON SCHOOL OF CLASSICAL HOMEOPATHY**
94 Green Dragon Lane
Winchmore Hill
London N21 2NJ
Tel:020 8360 8757

**PURTON HOUSE SCHOOL OF HOMEOPATHY**
Purton House
Purton Lane
Farnham Royal
Buckinghamshire SL2 3LY
Tel: 01753 646625

**THE SCHOOL OF HOMEOPATHY**
8 Kiln Road
Llanfoist
Abergavenny
Monmouthshire NP7 9NS
Tel: 01873 858962

## SPECIALIST HOMEOPATHIC PHARMACIES

**THE APOTHECARY**
Morthern Road Surgery
Rotherham
S. Yorks S66 1EU
Tel: 01709 531177
Website:
www.apothecary.co.uk

**AINSWORTH HOMEOPATHIC PHARMACY**
38 New Cavendish Street
London W1M 7LH
Tel: 020 7935 5330
Website:
www.ainsworth.com

**BUXTON AND GRANT**
176 Whiteladies Road
Bristol BS8 2XU
Tel: 0117 735025

**FREEMAN'S HOMEOPATHIC PHARMACY**
20 Main Street
Busby
Glasgow G76 8DU
Tel: 0141 644 1165
Website:
www.freechem.co.uk

**GALEN HOMEOPATHICS**
Lewell Mill
West Stafford
Dorchester
Dorset DT2 8AN
Tel: 01305 263996/265759

**HELIOS HOMEOPATHIC PHARMACY**
97 Camden Road
Tunbridge Wells
Kent TH1 2QP
Tel: 01892 537254
Website: www.helios.co.uk

**NELSON'S HOMEOPATHIC PHARMACY**
73 Duke Street
London W1M 6BY
Tel: 020 7629 3118
Website:
www.nelsons.co.uk

**WELEDA (UK) LTD**
Heanor Road
Ilkeston
Derbyshire DE7 8DR
Tel: 0115 930 9319
Website:
www.weleda.co.uk

*Homeopathic Registers, registers of practitioners are available from the professional organisations listed above.*

## INTERNET

**BOIRON LABORATORIES**
www.boiron.com

**THE EUROPEAN AND INTERNATIONAL COUNCILS FOR CLASSICAL HOMEOPATHY**
www.gn.apc.org/ecch.icch

**EUROPEAN COMMITTEE FOR HOMEOPATHY**
homeopathyeurope.org

**GLASGOW HOMEOPATHIC LIBRARY**
www.xcy76.dial.pipex.com
*Associated with the Glasgow Homeopathic Hospital, it has articles and research information available.*

**THE HOMEOPATHIC INFORMATION SERVICE**
www.hominf.org.uk
*Contains a Cured Symptoms Database, the full text of new provings and articles about provings.*

**HOMEOPATHIC INTERNET RESOURCES LIST (HOMEOWEB)**
www2.antenna.nl/homeoweb/resource.html

**INTERNATIONAL HOMEOPATHIC MEDICAL ORGANISATION**
www.rccm.org.uk
*Research Council for Complementary Medicine*

## WEBSITES OF GENERAL INTEREST

www.homeopathyhome.com

www.demystify.com

www.drlockie.com

www.homeopathy-uk.com

## JOURNALS

**BRITISH HOMEOPATHIC JOURNAL**
Faculty of Homeopathy
15 Clerkenwell Close
London EC1R 0AA
www.stockton-press.co.uk

**THE HOMEOPATH**
www.thehomeopath.ndirect.co.uk
*Journal of the Society of Homeopaths*

**EUROPEAN HOMEOPATHY (MÉDITIONS GROUP)**
1–3 rue du Départ
75014 Paris
France
Tel: 00 331 40 64 00 75

**HOMEOPATHY ONLINE**
www.lyghtforce.com/homeopathyonline

**TANTALUS, A JOURNAL OF BIOLUMANETICS**
www.biolumanetics.net/tantalus

# Further reading

## Reference works

Samuel Hahnemann, *Exposition of the Homeopathic Medical Doctrine or Organon of the Healing Art* 1856. Hahnemann's major work in which he presents the basis of his theory.

Dr Samuel Hahnemann, trans J. Kunzli, A. Naude, P. Pendleton, *The Organon of Medicine*, Tarcher Publications, Los Angeles, USA, 1982

## Medica materia

These works, used by homeopathic practitioners, list the homeopathic medicines, presenting the symptoms and modalities of each one.

Drs W. Boericke, Boericke & Tafel, *Pocket Manual of Homeopathic Materia Medica*, 9th edition, Philadelphia, USA, 1927

Dr Jacques Jouanny, Dr Denis Demarque, Dr Bernard Poitevin and Dr Yves Saint Jean, *Pharmacology and Homeopathic Materia Medica*, CEDH, 1995

Dr O.A. Julian, trans Virginia Mundy, *Materia Medica of New Homeopathic Remedies*, Beaconsfield Publishers, Beaconsfield, UK, 1979

## Overviews

These books address the history and development of homeopathy.

Blackie, Margery, *The Challenge of Homeopathy*, Unwin Hyman, London, 1981

Dr Marjory Blackie, eds., Dr Charles Elliot, Dr Frank Johnson, *Classical Homeopathy*, Beaconsfield Publishers, Beaconsfield, UK, 1986

Coulter, Harris L, *Homeopathic Science and Modern Medicine: The Physics of Healing with Microdoses*, North Atlantic Books, Berkeley, California, USA,1987

Ullman, Dana, *Homeopathy:Medicine for the 21st Century*, North Atlantic Books, Berkeley, California, USA, 1968

Vithoulkas, George, *Homeopathy: Medicine of the New Man*, Thorsons, 1985

## Practical Works

These books present the principles of homeopathy and offer an introduction.

Castro, Miranda, *The Complete Homeopathy Handbook*, Macmillan, 1990

Gaier, Harold, *Thorson's Encyclopedic Dictionary of Homeopathy*, Thorsons, 1991

Lockie, Andrew, *The family guide to homeopathy: the safe form of medicine for the future*, 1998

Dr Barry Rose, Dr Christina Scott-Montcrieff, *Homeopathy for Women*, Collins and Brown, 1998

Vithoulkas, George, *The Science of Homeopathy*, Thorsons, 1986

## Illustrated Works

Illustrated books which present homeopathy and its medicines.

Hammond, Christopher, *The Complete Family Guide to Homeopathy: an illustrated encyclopedia of safe and effective remedies*, 1995

Dr Andrew Lockie, Dr Nicola Geddes, *Homeopathy, The Principles and Practice of Treatment*, Dorling Kindersley, 1995

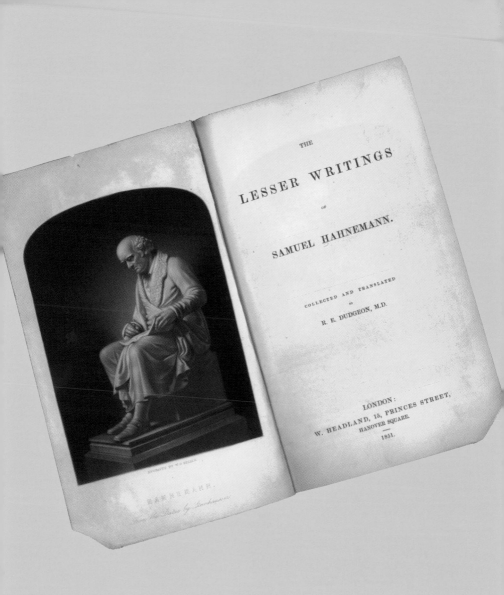

THE

# LESSER WRITINGS

OF

## SAMUEL HAHNEMANN.

COLLECTED AND TRANSLATED
BY
R. E. DUDGEON, M.D.

LONDON:
W. HEADLAND, 15, PRINCES STREET,
HANOVER SQUARE.
1851.

## ALLOPATHY

The term comes from the Greek *allos*, which means 'other', and *pathos*, meaning 'illness', and is used in contrast with the term homeopathy. It refers to orthodox medicine which views the body as made up of separate parts and systems and prescribes symptomatically.

## CINCHONA

While translating a text about cinchona bark, from which quinine is made, Hahnemann had the idea of testing it on himself, a healthy person, in order to understand how it worked. He noticed that cinchona produced in him the effects that he was supposed to be treating. Thus the idea of similarity was born.

## CONSTITUTION

The sum of the patient's reactions, susceptibility to, and way of manifesting, an illness.

## CONSTITUTIONAL REMEDY

A single remedy that can treat all an individual's ailments by correcting his imbalances at the deepest level.

## CONSTITUTIONAL TYPE

All the physical, mental and emotional characteristics of the patient which enable the homeopathic practitioner to work out which is the best remedy.

## DIATHESIS

There are four diatheses: tuberculinic, syphilitic, sycotic, psoric. (See page 71.) The term miasm is often used instead of diathesis.

## DILUTION

Homeopathic medicines are diluted to an infinitesimal degree to avoid all risk of toxicity and to seek the smallest effective dose. In centesimal dilutions, one drop of product is mixed with 99 drops of solvent to obtain a dilution of 1 c. Then, to one drop of this mixture is added 99 drops of solvent which produces a dilution of 2 c, and so on. Decimal dilutions are obtained by adding one drop of product to 9 drops of solvent (1D), and so on.

## DOSE

Homeopathic medicines can be bought in small phials. One pill is taken and can be repeated depending on the symptom response.

## DOUBLE BLIND

A method of testing drugs in which two groups of patients are randomly assigned to take either a drug or a placebo. Neither patients nor researchers know which group has taken which substance until the trial is over.

## GALENIC

All the different pharmaceutical forms in which the remedies are produced (granules, globules, ointments, gels, drops, essence, suppositories), a term relating to Galen, an Ancient Roman physician.

## GLOBULES

Small lactose balls impregnated with a homeopathic dilution. These may also be called pillules.

## HOMEOPATHY

The term comes from the Greek *homoios*, which means 'like', and *pathos*, which means 'suffering/disease'. It is thus a type of medical treatment using a substance that is similar to the illness.

## IMPREGNATION

Homeopathic medicines are made by spraying dilution onto lactose balls, which are therefore impregnated from the outside. This is distinct from allopathic medicines, in which the active substance is covered by an outer coating.

## INDICATION

A symptom suggesting certain treatment.

## IN VIVO

In vivo studies are carried out on people carrying an illness (as opposed to studying bacteria in a laboratory). Their purpose is to check the validity and measure the results of new treatments.

## IN VITRO

In vitro experiments are carried out in the laboratory on living cells. They enable biological and biochemical processes to be understood and explained.

## INDIVIDUALISATION

One of the basic principles of homeopathy: it is the patient not the disease that is treated. The treatment is tailored to the individual, taking into account his unique presentation of symptoms.

## INFINITESIMAL

A basic principle of homeopathy. Dilutions are so small that, according to classical chemistry, there is no longer any material trace of the main active constituent remaining. Homeopathy therefore acts according to a principle which seems more at home in the realm of physics. It is as if a 'message' is transmitted from the original substance to the solvent in which it is diluted.

## MATERIA MEDICA

Latin for 'materials of medicine' and meaning a reference work that lists the curative indications and therapeutic actions of homeopathic medicines. Initially put together by Hahnemann and his successors, the first Materia medica pura, composed of 6 volumes, appeared between 1811 and 1821.

## MIASM

In its strict sense, the term refers to the products emanating from a decomposing body (animal or vegetable). It is generally used to describe a chronic disease state resulting from infection or inherited effects. See also diathesis.

## MOTHER TINCTURE

The first stage in the medicine's manufacture which consists of steeping the substance (animal, vegetable or mineral) in a solvent, generally a mixture of alcohol and water, for several weeks. The liquid thus produced is then used to manufacture the different pharmaceutical forms.

## PATHOGENESIS

In homeopathy, all the physical and psychological symptoms developed by a healthy subject on whom a homeopathic substance is tried out.

## PLACEBO

A neutral substance (distilled water or sugar), used in double blind experiments to test the effectiveness of medicines.

## POTENTISATION

A process involving dilution and succussion to release and increase the medicinal power of a substance.

## REPERTORY

An index of the homeopathic Materia Medica by symptom. A list of remedies is indicated for each symptom. All modern day repertories use Kent's Repertory as their starting point.

## SIMILARS

This is the first basic principle of homeopathy: treat 'like with like', give the patient a product which produces in a healthy person the same symptoms shown by the patient.

## SUCCUSSION

The process of shaking the homeopathic medicine vigorously at each stage of manufacture.

## SUSCEPTIBILITY

The individual's sensitivity to a certain illness or his susceptibility to a particular remedy.

## TOXICITY

Homeopathy is completely non-toxic. It is administered in such low doses that it has no harmful side effects.

## TRITURATION

This process consists of grinding non-soluble substances in a mortar with lactose, until a powder is produced. This can be dissolved in a solvent, enabling a first dilution to be obtained.

# Contents

## Fact ⟩⟩ 2–12
Fun facts and quick quotes

## Discover ⟩⟩ 13–46

| | |
|---|---|
| Medical colleges and training: from theory ... | 15 |
| ... to practice | 15 |
| Should the symptoms always be confronted? | 16 |
| Apis or cortisone? | 19 |
| Like treats like | 19 |
| Hahnemann's frustration | 20 |
| The initial discovery | 23 |
| The theory of dilution | 24 |
| *Materia Medica* | 27 |
| 'Blind' testing | 28 |
| The world of the infinitely small | 31 |
| Homeopathy can be used to treat animals | 31 |
| The development of clinical trials | 32 |
| Homeopathy in laboratory tests | 35 |
| How does it work? | 36 |
| What remains of Hahnemann's discoveries? | 39 |
| The spread of a new therapy | 39 |
| The availability of homeopathic medicines | 43 |
| Homeopathy is a type of medicine which respects the individual | 44 |
| Homeopathy is the therapy of the future | 46 |

## Look ⟩⟩ 47–64
The manufaturing process – images from a homeopathic laboratory

# In practice ⟫ 65–96

| | |
|---|---|
| Like treats like | 66–67 |
| Constitution and identifying constitutional types | 68–69 |
| Temperament and diathesis | 70–71 |
| The manufacture of homeopathic medicines | 72–73 |
| The potencies | 74–75 |
| Actions and reactions | 76–77 |
| The homeopathic consultation | 78–79 |
| Allopathy and homeopathy | 80–81 |
| Homeopathy – working with other therapies | 82–83 |
| Self-medication and treating a child | 84–85 |
| Treating an adult | 86–87 |
| Treating an elderly person | 88–89 |
| Treating an animal | 90–91 |
| The ten basic homeopathic medicines | 92–93 |
| Types of homeopathic medicine | 94–95 |
| Homeopathy across the globe | 96 |

# Find out ⟫ 97–125

| | |
|---|---|
| Water has a memory | 98–101 |
| Homeopathy's key dates | 102–103 |
| Which homeopathic remedy profile fits you? | 104–107 |
| The homeopathic family medicine chest | 108–109 |
| Ten common ailments and their treatments | 110–111 |
| How to find a good homeopath | 112–113 |
| Generally accepted ideas: true or false? | 114–115 |
| Homeopathy statistics | 116–117 |
| Information and training | 118–121 |
| Further reading | 122–123 |
| Glossary | 124–125 |

# Important notice for the reader

# Credits

**P14,** Aspe Valley, plate G.Lopez, Bios – **P17,** *A Convalescent*, painting by Frank Holl, The Bridgeman Art Library – **P18**, Apis mellifica, Bios. – **P21,** *The Apothicary*, plate Jean–Loup Charmet – **P22,** Portrait of Hahnemann, plate Boiron; China, plate Montpellier Faculty of Medicine – **P25** *Edward Jenner's first vaccination against cowpox in 1796*, painting by Gaston Mélingue, plate Jean–Loup Charmet – **P26,** plate C. Mure/Boiron –**P29,** *Homeopathic doctors*, caricature by Daumier, plate Jean–Loup Charmet – **P30,** plate C. Mure/Boiron – **P33,** plate Pierrot – **P34** plate INSERM – **P37,** plate Bill Longcore/Explorer – **P38,** Laurel and Hardy, plate MGM – **P42,** plate C Mure/Boiron –

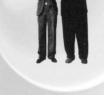

**P45,** plate Y. Geoffray/Boiron – **P46,** plate PG Lombard/Boiron – **P48–49,** plate Y. Geoffray/Boiron – **P50–51,** plate PG Lombard/Boiron – **P488–49,** plate Y Geoffray/Boiron – **P50–51,** plate PG Lombard/Boiron – **P52,** plate V Burger–Phanie/Boiron – **P53,** plate V Burger–Phanie/Boiron – **P54,** plate Boiron, **P55,** plate C. Mure/Boironn – **P56–57,** plate Boiron –**P.58,** plate P. Maisonneuve/Dolisos – **P.59,** plate H Bigot/Boiron – **P60,** plate Y Geoffray/Boiron – **P.61,** plate P Maisonneuve/Dolisos – **P62,** plate V. Burger–Phanie/Boiron – **P63,** plate Y. Geoffray/Boiron – **P.64,** plate BSIP Chassenet – **P.66 to 96,** Idé computer graphics – **P98 to 125,** illustrations: Philippe Gaulier – **P.123,** Homeopathic Library, Glasgow.

# Acknowledgements

The authors and editors would like to thank Dr Sarembaud for his careful re–reading, the Boiron Laboratories and in particular Ms Bénédicte Sanimorte and Corine Mure for their help and assistance with the illustrations and their comments on the texts; Anne Sebbag of Similia publishing and Emmanuel Brambilla of the Dolisos Laboratories, as well as Dr Jacqueline Pecker, veterinary surgeon, for their help in producing this work.

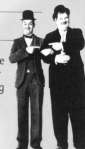